My Action Plan
For Stopping the Symptoms of
Mitral Valve Prolapse
Syndrome/Dysautonomia

Including the Overlapping Symptoms of
POTS, Fibromyalgia and
Chronic Fatigue Syndrome/ME

By
Joan Anderson

GW00646731

Joan Anderson Communications, LLC
For more information, visit
www.MVPSBook.com

Library of Congress Cataloging-in-Publication Data
First printing, October 2021

ISBN's: 979-8-9850668-0-7 (e-book)   979-8-9850668-1-4 (paperback)

Disclaimer

The information in this book is not intended to diagnose, treat, or cure any disease. This book is not a substitute for quality healthcare provided by a licensed and knowledgeable healthcare practitioner.

The author and publisher are not providing or recommending medical, psychological or any other kind of personal or professional services in this book and expressly disclaim all responsibility for any injury, damage, negative consequences or loss that the reader may incur as a consequence of following the information detailed in this book.

Instead, this book explains how, with the help of many healthcare professionals and extensive research, the author developed her action plan. The content is solely the opinion of the author as it pertains to her own personal medical and health needs.

This book is designed to explain the processes and methods used to research and learn about the author's personal health issues. The information contained in this, or any other documents, should not be construed as a claim or representation that any procedure or product mentioned, including supplements and homeopathic remedies, constitutes a specific treatment or cure, palliative, or ameliorative for any condition.

The author does not recommend nor endorse any specific test, physician, product, procedure, opinion or any other information provided in this book. Nor does the author recommend to others any of the treatments she uses for herself. Each person's health and medical situation is different. When the word "you" is used, it does not refer to the reader but is used in the universal or generic sense of "people in general" as opposed to the more formal word, "one."

References are provided for informational purposes only and do not constitute an endorsement of any websites or other sources. Readers should be aware that the sites listed in this book may change. Research about this subject is ongoing and subject to conflicting interpretations.

While every effort has been made to provide accurate information, the author and publisher cannot be held responsible for any errors or omissions. Before making any decisions based on the information found in this book, a person should first check with his or her physician. To protect the identities of the people whose actions or stories appear in this book, no names have been used, and in some cases, the author created composites.

Some of the information in the book is based on, to the best of the author's recall, discussions with doctors and other people with MVPS or writings of other people with MVPS as well as on her research notes and experiences. Conclusions regarding all this information, which may be noted in this book, are based on the author's personal opinion as it relates to her situation specifically and her health and medical issues.

The author is not a doctor. She is a person who was diagnosed with mitral valve prolapse. The information in this book is intended to share her treatment experiences, her opinions and research methods and how MVPS has affected her. In a medical emergency, call 911 immediately

Dedication

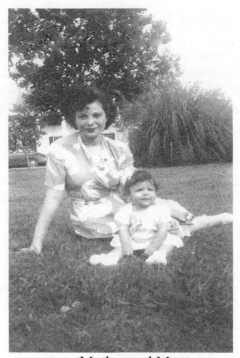

Mother and Me

This book is dedicated to my mother,
who suffered all her life with the many symptoms of
mitral valve prolapse syndrome but was never diagnosed.
I did not know. I did not understand. Now I do.

Acknowledgments

Welcome to the World of MVPS, Dorothy Sanders!

She never knew there was such a thing as mitral valve prolapse syndrome until she met me. Though she had no background in the medical field and was puzzled by how often a healthy, young person like me would fall ill, she was always respectful and concerned and never questioned or doubted my condition.

Dorothy, my dear friend and writing partner for more than thirty-five years, has seen all my highs and lows, driven me to several ER visits and brought me home from the hospital more than once. She worried with me when I was given erroneous but frightening diagnoses and comforted me as she saw me struggle with the litany of symptoms she had never seen in one person.

We learned to work around MVPS and become productive writers. We both worked in the news field and together turned our abilities to writing scripts for the stage.

We did a series for the Prevention Players, a kickoff for community health education seminars, and were at times the opening act for other educational programs. And then, of course, we wrote for fun with comedies that were produced on stages across the United States. These projects lighten the heart and always left me feeling better. We worked well together. And I am lucky to have had her as a friend and co-writer. Talented and creative, Dorothy held a master's degree from Harvard and a PhD from Texas Woman's University. Her many years in the education field, both in the classroom and as a consultant, always elevated our work materials.

When I decided to write the book on my life with MVPS, she was right there to help me and to work with me as we have always done. Her editing abilities have been invaluable in helping me shape the organization, content and clarity of this book. I am so grateful that she prodded me to write this book when life and other responsibilities took my attention from what she knew was an important project for me to accomplish. She was right. Writing this book has been a challenging but cathartic experience, but most of all has shown me how far I have come in creating a higher level of health that I thought MVPS would never allow me to find. Thank you, Dorothy, for living through it with me and helping me document it.

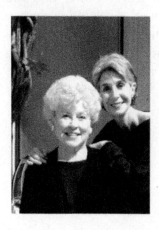

Note

My dear friend Dorothy Sanders passed away unexpectedly in January 2021. My sadness has not yet lifted as I finalize this book. She worked with me every step of the way to help keep me motivated and on track. I am so pleased that she knew I had finished it and put it in the capable hands of Rana K. Williamson, PhD, for final editing. Thank you, Dorothy, for your encouragement and support and for enriching my life in so many ways. You are dearly missed.

Thank You Rana!

If you find this book easy to read and well-formatted with documentations just a click away, it is because my friend, Rana K. Williamson, PhD, agreed to edit it.

A former university history instructor, Rana took the time (a lot of time) to help me get this book to fruition. She did this even while working on her own projects—the highly successful Jinx Hamilton series. She and her writing partner, Patricia Pauletti, publish their best-selling books under the pen name Juliette Harper.

This enthralling series merges influences of *Harry Potter* and Jim Butcher's *The Dresden Files* to craft an enchanting urban paranormal fantasy experience readers say they just can't put down! Thank you, Rana. I could not have done it without you. Looking forward to reading the books in your next series.

TABLE OF CONTENTS

Foreword

Let's imagine. You are feeling something you've never felt before. Maybe it's pain. Maybe it's a fluttering in your heart. Or it could be something in your gut that makes you double over.

A 200-million-year-old device in your brain will react. It's your amygdala. I'm calling it a device because it doesn't think. It just reacts. The amygdala monitors what is going on inside you and outside you. If what is happening has happened before, it's "Ho, hum. Been there. Done that." The amygdala ignores it. But if it senses something you haven't experienced before, it releases stress hormones. Why? Something different could be life-threatening.

The reason the amygdala has been around for 200 million years is its success. By ignoring the familiar and reacting to the unfamiliar, it has helped preserve the lives of the creatures equipped with it. One of the first creatures to have an amygdala was the Tyrannosaurus rex. A T-rex wasn't very smart. That massive reptile had a brain the size of a German shepherd.

A T-rex survived as long as it did because whenever anything unfamiliar happened, its amygdala released stress hormones that caused an urge to run.

Since a T-rex didn't have enough brainpower to distinguish a life-threatening emergency from a false alarm, it just ran away.

Better safe than sorry.

Fast forward to now. You inherited this device. It's no smarter than it was 200 million years ago. Any unexpected pain or physical sensations will cause your amygdala to release stress hormones. The stress hormones do the same thing in you that they did in the T-rex. They create the urge to escape. If escape routes are blocked, the urge is redirected to fight.

But with the threat inside your body, you can't escape it. Nor can you fight it. Trapped, you may panic. You have intelligence the T-rex didn't have. But in a state of panic, your reptile brain takes over. Let's say someone gets you to an ER. There, your challenge is to set your reptile brain aside. Otherwise, you will not be able to use your high-level thinking to team up with your doctors. Even though you are extremely revved up, you need to down regulate well enough to offer them the best source of information available: what you are feeling, where you are feeling it, how did it start, and how long has it been going on.

Did you ever take a pet to a vet? Think about it. Your dog or cat can't tell the vet where it hurts. Your vet is shooting in the dark. Even if it is your pet parrot, what the parrot says won't be helpful. Your doctors need you to give them the information they need. But how can you downregulate the feeling of alarm enough to team up with your doctors and potentially save your life? Frankly, unless you have programmed your subcortex to automatically attenuate your feelings of alarm, you won't be able to.

In a state of panic, your conscious mind is overwhelmed. Anything you do consciously only adds to the feeling of being overwhelmed. You could wait 90 seconds for the stress hormones to burn off. But as they burn off, awareness of what may be a life-threatening emergency will replace the stress hormones you burn with more stress hormones. So how can you keep your wits about you? You can do it the same way firefighters, law enforcement, and ER personnel do it. You train your mind in advance to deal with the situation. This is because, in a life-threatening situation, we do not "rise to the occasion." Rather we descend to the level of our training.

It is essential that you train your unconscious procedural memory (it still works in a crisis because it is in the subcortex) to activate the only system that can override the effect the stress hormones are having on you: the parasympathetic nervous system. Para means against. When activated, the parasympathetic nervous system works against the sympathetic nervous system, the system that is pushing you into panic

You need to train your unconscious procedural memory to automatically activate your parasympathetic nervous system when needed. Once it is activated, your parasympathetic nervous system overrides your reptile brain's fight-or-flight response. This allows your high-level thinking to function. Without automatic activation of the parasympathetic, in a life-threatening situation, we can be our own worst enemy. When hyperaroused, we no longer separate what is real from

what is imaginary. What we fear becomes our reality. We are sure the worst outcome is inevitable. This renders us unable to give accurate information about our condition to those who are trying to help.

In this book, Joan Anderson shares her action plan for dealing with health choices. At some time in your life, you will face a situation that may be life-threatening. She shows you how she teamed up with medical professions who earnestly wanted to help her. She reveals how she identifies and chooses the doctors who would be the best for her team.

Joan will tell you how she learned about various tests, including diagnostic imaging where she found a method to get a better definition for her thyroid issue while avoiding radiation. She will tell you how she, as a patient, can advocate for something better and how others can choose to do it too.

Joan details how she determines which medication options to accept and which to reject. After reading this book, you may want to develop a plan too, specific for you, to do the same.

What I hope to contribute to Joan's book is how to train your mind in advance to handle a crisis in a cool, calm, collected, rational, and effective manner. If you can present your medical history and your present self-observations accurately, you will be your doctor's best source of information. To do this, you need to be able, even in a crisis, to keep your high-level thinking working. After all, isn't that when you need your high-level thinking most?

One last word. And this is personal. A few years ago, my wife, Marie, had a stroke. Initially, the right side of her body was paralyzed. Now she can get around with a walker. Her stroke was completely preventable. If she had had the information in this book, she could have avoided the stroke, and our life together now would be very different. Read this book.

Captain Tom Bunn, LCSW, Author of Panic Free, The 10-Day Program to End Panic, Anxiety, and Claustrophobia and Founder of The SOAR Program for nervous flyers

The Diagnosis

A Benign Click

The author has no underlying structural or functional problems with her heart. She was diagnosed with mitral valve prolapse when a physician listened to her heart and noted a benign click as the mitral valve closed. The author has what is called mitral valve prolapse syndrome/dysautonomia, a problem with the autonomic nervous system and not the heart.

The Author's MVPS Medical History

I Have Walked in Your Shoes

Duh-duh-dum! My experience with MVPS began with a rapid but mild flutter in my chest and has since dragged me to the gates of hell. A few minutes after that first faint sensation, the flutter happened again. I sat up in bed and the feeling stopped. The next night when I lay down, the same thing occurred.

I wasn't particularly worried about these gentle flutters, but I had never felt them before. I mentioned the sensation to my doctor on my next visit.

I was thirty-one years old and in good health.

The flutters had become an almost nightly occurrence. I would lie down, and then the fluttering would start.

I would sit up, and the feeling stopped.

The doctor listened to my heart and found nothing wrong. He surmised that the accumulation of caffeine in my system from four daily cups of coffee was responsible for the flutters. The quiet of night made the sensations more noticeable. That made sense. I eliminated coffee from my diet, but the flutters continued.

Every time I saw a doctor, whether for my well-woman examination or for a cold or flu, I mentioned the fluttering. Each time the doctor listened to my heart and heard nothing. My heartbeat was strong and normal. But I had nagging questions. If the flutters were nothing, why wouldn't they go away? If the sensation was normal, why hadn't I felt it throughout my life?

Finding a Specialist

An internist, who had been my doctor several years earlier, closed his general practice to specialize in cardiology. I made an appointment with him. As I drove to his office, I began to have doubts. I felt great and hadn't felt any fluttering in days.

I checked in with the receptionist and looked around the waiting room. I was a thirty-one-year-old, healthy woman in a room filled with extremely sick older people. My doubts grew. Did I really need to see a cardiologist? I did not know that this was only the beginning of a lifetime of doubts and confusion revolving around my mitral valve prolapse symptoms.

The First Diagnosis

Surprisingly, the doctor took me seriously at a time when heart disease was considered a problem for men, not women. After asking me a round of typical cardiac questions, he pulled out his stethoscope and listened to my chest. He took his time. No one else had listened to my heart that carefully. He asked me to stand up and slowly squat down and stand back up again while he listened. I did this several times while his stethoscope moved across my chest and then my back.

"I heard a click," he said. "You have mitral valve prolapse." I had never heard of the condition before. I was relieved when he told me that the relatively benign disorder did not require medical treatment except a course of antibiotics before dental and surgical procedures as a precaution against the low risk of an infection in the heart called endocarditis.

He told me that he was seeing more people with MVP but that most had no symptoms. Then he scheduled an echocardiogram that

18

confirmed his opinion. My valve was billowing but closing completely, and there was no regurgitation or blood backing up.

Fifteen Years Later

That mild and innocuous fluttering that my doctor said was no cause for concern would, fifteen years later, usher in an array of frightening symptoms. They terrorized my body, attacked my spirit, dictated my life choices and sent me to the doctor more times than I could count—and to the hospital on more than one occasion. No one told me about the "*syndrome.*" I didn't even know

I had it until, without warning, a sledgehammer hit me that, at times, literally took my breath away.

The Symptoms Begin with a Vengeance

During one of the happiest and healthiest periods of my life, MVPS insidiously reared its head. I was working as an administrator for a hospital health system. I loved my job and was enjoying a high level of professional success. Then one day, while reading the newspaper, I noticed my right arm, which I was using to hold one side of the paper open, was tingling and feeling weak.

I put down the paper and rested my arm, but the weird feeling remained. I decided to go to the clinic to see my doctor, who ordered a head CAT (CT) scan to determine if there was any brain damage indicating a stroke. I was fine and was told that I was having a migraine aura headache.

Then one night, out of the blue, intense chest pain awakened me. A few seconds passed before I could even comprehend what I felt. It was an incredibly stressful time for me. There were extra pressures at work and home, but I knew I shouldn't ignore chest pain.

I went to the emergency room at the hospital where I worked. They took good care of me and ran tests to rule out a cardiac event. The diagnosis pointed to upper stomach issues as the cause of the pain. I went home relieved.

After that, I started having nagging low back pain that intensified until I couldn't even lift my purse. Muscle relaxants and pain pills didn't help. The problem evolved into sciatic nerve pain. I couldn't walk more than a few steps without excruciating pain.

I had never been so incapacitated. Diagnosed with a bulging disk, I spent more than a month in bed. Just as surgery was looking inevitable, acupuncture put me back on my feet.

Not long afterward, I had minor surgery that, because of a small complication, sent me back into the operating room only hours later.

The double anesthetic and surgery took a tremendous toll that delayed my recovery. Later I realized this incident along with my back problem had aggravated my MVPS symptoms.

The Stress Test Debacle

Before my surgery, I took a stress test because I was having mild, occasional chest pain. The test results showed a false positive. The electrical readings from the EKG indicated a significant arterial blockage. When the doctor stopped the treadmill and told me, fear shot through me.

I was quickly laid on the exam table for an echocardiogram. The doctor watched the monitor to see if my blood flow was indeed impaired. I waited, still hooked up to the EKG leads. I was breathless, panting from the fear and from my workout on the treadmill.

Moments later, the cardiologist casually said, "No, you're fine. The echocardiogram shows a normal flow. It was a false positive. You're perfectly fine to undergo surgery."

I also had a false positive on two other occasions that left me doubting the validity of the stress test.

How could I trust the results either way? My doctor told me that a false positive still leaves a 15%-20% error rate. That means that there is still a 15%-20% chance that the stress test is correct and a problem does exist.

So, which is right? Since I consistently had false-positive stress tests and I was having mild chest pains, a dark cloud of doubt hovered over me. I decided I would never do a stress test without an accompanying echocardiogram to confirm the results.

More Chest Pains

I was glad to know my heart was stable and strong during both my surgeries, but that bit of comfort didn't last long. Only six weeks later, the chest pain returned with greater force. I rushed to the hospital where I worked. After running all the typical cardiac tests, the doctors diagnosed acid indigestion again and sent me home.

Tired but relieved, I went to work the next day only to be called by the head of the emergency medicine department that afternoon. All EKGs administered in the ER are routinely reviewed by other doctors. The physician who went over my EKG saw some irregularities and recommended that I follow up with my cardiologist. Panicked, I called the office and was told I could come right in.

The cardiologist's office was across the street from mine, so I was there in minutes. He ran another EKG that was also irregular. Although he did not think the results indicated a serious problem, he told me that the only way to be sure was to do a cardiac catheterization.

During the procedure, a thin tube is inserted in an artery or vein and threaded through the blood vessels to the heart. This allows the doctor to find and sometimes treat any problems. The cardiologist sent me home to consider that option.

The Cardiac Catheterization

The choice wasn't an easy one. I didn't want to do a cardiac catheterization, but since the chest pains continued, not knowing wasn't a risk I wanted to take either. The luxury of choice became irrelevant, however, when, several days later, I awakened in the middle of the night with another round of intense pain.

I went to the emergency room again and was admitted. After much discussion, I agreed to undergo the cardiac catheterization, which was performed that day. Although heavily sedated, I was awake throughout the entire procedure.

After what seemed like only minutes, the doctor told me that I was okay. There were no blockages. I left the hospital relieved but feeling battered from all the procedures. I felt emotionally and physically drained. It was an omen of what was to come.

MVPS Gets Nasty

Over the next few months, MVPS took over my life and my health. One symptom after another pounded my body, leaving me terrified and bewildered. On any given day, I had one or more symptoms: migraines, dizziness, IBS flare-ups, reactions to food sensitivities, anxiety, hot flashes, arrhythmias and sensitivities to chemicals and fragrances. I was a mess and scared all the time.

I knew I had to do something to pull myself together, or I would continue in a downward spiral.

The cardiologist offered to give me a prescription for a beta blocker and an antianxiety drug. I declined and instead began a journey to find better answers on my own. Even when I felt too sick to work, I still forged forward, determined to regain control.

Diagnosing Myself

Researching a health issue was a natural path for me. I have worked in various areas of the healthcare field for most of my professional life. I was sure I could find effective treatments for my condition. But first, I had to find out what was wrong with me.

I left the hospital without a helpful diagnosis but with a basic clean bill of health. I also had a feeling of being somewhat patronized. This would later turn into outright disdain from one of the doctors I saw in the clinic.

Fortunately, the internet was coming into its own with lots of information available, so I didn't have to spend hours at the medical library. I began my search at home.

My inquiries regarding my symptoms led me to several MVPS sites. I was surprised. I didn't know that MVP could cause so many problems. But it was still a relief to know it was nothing more serious, even if it was an alarming departure from my past experiences with this disorder.

Finding a Treatment, Finding a Doctor—The Journey Begins

I spent hours on the internet reading everything I could find, including bulletin board postings from symptomatic patients whose experiences equaled or exceeded mine.

They were not dying, but they were not living well either. Almost all the postings I read were from people taking prescription drugs daily to try to control their symptoms.

These drugs included beta blockers, antidepressants, antianxiety medications, or a combination of them all. It did not appear that the people taking drugs who posted online were finding relief. When I studied the drugs and potential side effects, I learned that the medications were not necessarily a panacea for MVPS but instead could cause some of the same symptoms as MVPS or new symptoms. In light of my past problems tolerating drugs, the risk wasn't worth it.

Delaying or refusing cardiac or psychiatric drugs would not cause irreparable damage to me. MVPS is not considered life-threatening. These facts affirmed my decision to seek a nondrug route for symptom relief.

Today, I am significantly better. My health has noticeably improved, and for the most part, my symptoms are under control or gone. If a problem should occur, I have the tools to deal with it quickly and effectively. As a result, I am not at the mercy of MVPS symptoms. I am not living in fear or running to the ER. I am learning new information all the time that is helping me continue to improve.

This book began as treatment research notes. I wanted to be able to refer to the pertinent information I had found during a flare-up. Now that I have compiled my notes into a book with my memories, experiences and professional input, this volume serves as my action plan to remind me of the treatments I have found that have been helpful to me.

Part I
How I Developed My Personal Action Plan

Chapter 1
This Book Is
My Personal MVPS Action Plan

What I Do to Prevent and Stop the Symptoms

I promised myself not to accept the limits of my doctors or the medical system and to never stop searching for better answers. In this book, I document my findings and the approach I use to stay as safe and healthy as possible. The action plan helps me to remember what I have learned and gives me a place to run during an MVPS emergency.

I Want to Be Prepared

When I board a plane or close a hotel room door, I always look at the escape route. If there is a fire or an emergency, I don't want to be at the mercy of panic. I want to be prepared. This is why schools have fire drills.

I feel the same way when MVPS symptoms strike out

of the blue. Fear and adrenaline put me in a fight-or-flight mode, which compromises my judgment. I want and need to be thoughtful, calm and in control.

Who is in Control, Me or My Lizard Brain?

The primitive portion of the brain, the amygdala, sometimes referred to as the "Lizard" brain, handles basic body function and is in charge of the fight-or-flight response which sends adrenaline racing through the body. Without a plan, I am at the mercy of this part of the brain. The fight-or-flight response can save a person by allowing them to react quickly without thinking, but I want to override that reaction when dealing with MVPS symptoms. (See: *Psychology Today*, "Your Lizard Brain.")

My symptoms have never signaled an emergency, and there are actions I can take to alleviate them. If I can't be calm in the moment to deal effectively with the symptom, I want to consider decisions that I made when I *was* calm and thinking clearly.

The medical staffs in the emergency room don't panic since they have been trained to act effectively in the face of critical issues. That takes planning. That's what I've done. Self-training helps me to make better decisions when I am in a reactive mode.

Under the influence of adrenaline, I forget that I have tools and treatments at my disposal to address non-life-threatening symptoms.

My original reference guide for crisis management comprises Part II of this book and details my MVPS Action Plan.

While exchanging information with a woman experiencing a significant MVPS flare-up, I realized my research might be of help to others. Though she was well-informed about many aspects of MVPS, the woman's fear and lack of a plan felt all too familiar to me.

At the end of our meeting, she thanked me and asked if my large folder of information represented notes for a book. I explained that I kept the material for my own reference needs. She said, "You really need to write a book. It would be so helpful." With my background working as a medical reporter, I found those words hard to ignore

This Is *My* Action Plan

In this book, I share the development of my plan and the 5 Patient Principles that were instrumental to my improvement. I offer this material as a sample from which readers can conduct their own treatment research relative to their preferences, unique medical needs, and in partnership with healthcare professionals.

The plan presented here is designed specifically for me and is based on my perspective, values, risk choices, physiology, and level of health. It emphasizes my most distressing MVPS symptoms. We may all have the same or similar diagnosis, but we are not the same. What works for me might not be right for you. Please read the disclaimer at the beginning of this book.

Chapter 2
How and Why I Developed
My MVPS Action Plan

That barely noticeable flutter that I first felt at age thirty-one ushered in a frightening array of future symptoms. Over the years, fear, confusion, and a sense of isolation undermined my ability to understand my body and made me more dependent on the medical system.

Even after I was diagnosed with MVPS, nothing changed. I was completely at the mercy of this "benign," often discounted and medically irrelevant disorder. At the onset, I was told MVPS posed nothing that should cause me any concern. Really? *Nothing?*

On My Own

At my worst, I was sick with what seemed like every symptom in the medical books and was scared I was dying. The doctors and ER staff did nothing to help. I had two choices.

- Take a variety of powerful psychiatric and cardiac drugs to cover the symptoms, as the doctors recommended, but risk drug side effects.
- Take control of my healthcare and look outside typical MVPS treatment options for safer and more effective answers.

I chose the second option.

Starting Over

I was on a fast-moving downward spiral. I thought life as I knew it was over. With nothing to lose and fear be damned, I dumped my cold, indifferent doctors and never looked back. Instead, I interviewed new physicians and found some helpful ones. Accustomed to intensive research as a medical reporter, I began investigating facts that were critical to my treatment.

New Approach

Looking outside mainstream conventional thinking about MVPS served me well. Many doors opened for me I never knew existed. I've read virtually everything available about MVPS. Most of the materials were invaluable. I'm grateful to everyone who shared their information. But what I found was not enough to get my symptoms under control.

There had to be more options. I kept looking and stayed open-minded. This approach helped me recover my life without cardiac and psychiatric drugs. With less dependence on the medical establishment, I gained more freedom and suffered less fear.

My Safety Net

But most importantly, I relied on something I developed and used as a reporter—my 5 Patient Principles. Those principles protected and guided me through the medical system. I knew I would need them to navigate the dark, scary place where MVPS had sent me. I had abandoned those principles for the false security of the medical system, but now I welcomed their return like an old friend. I will detail each of these principles and my use of them in Chapter 3.

Building My Action Plan

I instinctively knew that to develop an effective treatment plan I had to temporarily wipe the slate clean of everything I thought I knew about MVPS. Most of all, I had to take a fresh and unemotional look at my symptoms. I also needed to critically evaluate the pros and cons of the medical system as it related to MVPS. I began an intensive search for new information and treatments that could help me. I took copious notes on everything I found including the input from my new doctors.

Breaking the MVPS Symptom Code

My MVPS symptoms do not mean what I think they mean. They mimic serious health problems, causing my body to speak a foreign language. This breakdown in communications complicated everything.

I was running from doctor to doctor, and often to the emergency room, looking to experts to interpret confusing and scary symptoms. I wanted them to tell me I was okay or provide necessary medical attention. That useless pursuit wasn't working.

I had to learn how to better understand my body's signals. I searched for information, interventions and tools I could use at home to make sound decisions, assess my symptoms, and stop worrying.

Getting a better understanding of my body's language helped me target the actual problem and to determine when and where to seek a medical consultation. Understanding my body was paramount to finding answers and taking positive action.

Finding Doctors

I've seen the best and the worst of our medical system and everything in between. I've been discounted, made worse and deliberately attacked—but also received exceptional compassion in unexpected places. Each experience sent me farther down the road to finding better medical care.

Just because conventional medicine does not have the answers does not mean there are no answers to be found elsewhere.

Doctors know that there has been a significant economic shift in the past three decades. Patient healthcare dollars once spent on conventional medicine are now being spent on alternative and preventive services and products. Not all conventional doctors have come around, but the trend has more than started.

I have not seen doctors recognized as MVPS specialists, although I am aware of physicians in the field whose patients consider them to be kind and helpful. I have looked for a specific kind of physician. The physician who knows conventional medicine as well as nutrition and supplementation and who looks for the underlying cause of health problems, in my opinion, offers a powerful combination of options. This is especially true for the more informed, chronically ill patients like me, who are often referred to as "demanding" because they are desperately looking for something more helpful.

Patients who decide not to settle for less from their doctors form a powerful group that can improve the system for everyone. The medical industry can, and often does, respond to consumer demand.

I Stopped Looking for Answers in All the Wrong Places

Some doctors are, in my opinion, neither understanding nor helpful. The unsigned article, "What is Mitral Valve Prolapse Syndrome?" (mvpresource.com, 20 May 2013) offers a telling example of medical bias about MVPS.

While the site does have some useful information sprinkled throughout, I found opinions in it that I consider to be blatantly uninformed. Consider this excerpt:

"There is also a standard MVPS personality type, according to some experts. Patients tend to be nervous, anxious, compulsive individuals who talk fast, sleep too little, avoid taking medications and visit hospital emergency rooms more often than they need to."

The "traits" listed are symptoms. The site, offered as a resource to help people, offensively identifies a "personality trait" rather than accurately defining legitimate aspects of MVPS from which people like me suffer.

The notion that I have a personality trait that causes me to avoid medications is absurd. I get limited value out of most of the medications currently offered for MVPS treatment. Having suffered horrible side effects, I would say my refusal to use these drugs speaks to basic human survival instincts

Informed Doctors Know This

Consider the words of a physician with a better understanding of the condition.

"People with mitral valve prolapse are especially sensitive to all kinds of drugs and medications." (Ronald Hoffman, M.D. *Natural Therapies for Mitral Valve Prolapse*. New York: McGraw-Hill Education, 11 January 1999.)

My experience with such "experts" quoted in the article motivated me to go out on my own and take control of my healthcare. I don't want medical help from doctors who judge me by my symptoms, because they have little or nothing to offer me.

Finding My Best Answers in the Right Places

The books listed below were the most helpful to me and have endured the test of time. In my estimation, they are packed with the most useful information, and over the years, they have remained valuable to me.

Here is my short but top-rated book list.

1. Ronald Hoffman, M.D. *Natural Therapies for Mitral Valve Prolapse: A Good Health Guide. Keats Good Health Guides.* New York: McGraw Hill, 1 February 1999. A short, concise, and

comprehensive article by Dr. Hoffman is one of the best I've read explaining MVPS and its prevention. http://www.drhoffman.com

2. Cheryl and James F. Durante. *The Mitral Valve Prolapse Syndrome/Dysautonomia Survival Guide*. Oakland: New Harbinger Publications, 11 January 1999.

The Durantes founded the Society for MVP Syndrome, a group to which I belonged for many years until the organization dissolved. The society's newsletter, *The Beat*, gave me ongoing reassurance and valuable resources along with available seminars and videos. I have kept every copy. I am tremendously grateful, as I'm sure are others, for the enormous contribution made by the Durantes to our understanding of MVPS.

3. Tom Bunn. *Panic Free: The 10-Day Program to End Panic, Anxiety, and Claustrophobia.* Novato, California: New World Library, 30 April 2019. The best book I've found to teach readers how to stop adrenaline and escape the fear and symptoms the hormone causes.

I met the author on the phone—Captain Tom—in 2005 when I purchased his Fear of Flying course. A retired pilot and licensed therapist, he combined the best of several approaches to create a system that cured me of my fear when every other program failed.

His unique method, presented in this book, can also help people who suffer with general panic and anxiety issues. I will discuss this system at greater length later in this book, but here is more information about the book and the author from the publisher:

Panic, and its close cousins, anxiety and claustrophobia, have long been a problem without a reliable solution. In most cases, the estimated six million Americans who suffer with a panic disorder receive only marginal relief from psychotherapy, usually Cognitive Behavioral Therapy (CBT), medication, or the two combined. While CBT has been found to stop panic in only one of seven patients, the medications often added on to CBT are addictive, needed in high doses to combat panic, and involved in thirty percent of prescription drug overdose deaths.

After years of working to help sufferers, author Tom Bunn found a better way. His system uses the part of the brain that is not flooded with the stress hormones instead of the part that is and causes the panic. This "unconscious procedural memory" can be programmed to control panic by preventing the release of stress hormones and activating the parasympathetic nervous system. It sounds complicated but is not, requiring just ten days and no drugs or doctors. Panic Free: The 10-Day Program to End Panic, Anxiety, and Claustrophobia includes specific instructions for dealing with common panic triggers such as MRIs, bridges, airplane travel, and tunnels. Because panic is such a profoundly life-limiting problem, Bunn's technique is a true life-changer.

4. Al Davies, M.D. *Beatin' the Nomia.* (25 May 2013)

When I found Dr. Davies online in the 1990s, he seemed to be on the cutting edge of MVPS research and understanding. I purchased his first publication, *MVP Syndrome Patient Guide,* at a time when my symptoms had become problematic and frightening.

His position on dysautonomia was: "These patients are super sensitive to their own adrenaline and related hormones. What may make a normal person's heart rate rise by 10 beats per minute makes these patients' heart rates rise by 24, with pounding in the chest and an ominous sense of impending doom."

At the time, I found the Q&A section of his website with questions from people with MVP symptoms like mine. Dr. Davies' candid answers were informative, reassuring and comforting.

When I called his office at a Houston, Texas, university, Dr. Davies answered the phone himself. Although he was not accepting patients at the time, he spoke with me for almost an hour. He did not consult on my personal health issues but provided general information on MVPS that helped me sort out a great deal. I am still grateful for the time and expertise he shared.

At the time of this writing (late 2020), I could not find a website or locate a copy of his original *Patient Guide*. The book *Beatin' the Nomia!*, though somewhat dated, includes that helpful Q&A information.

The description of the book reads: *Beatin' the 'Normal! is a compendium for MVP Dysautonomia / POTS patients who need to understand its clinical spectrum and presentation, its physiological manifestations and biochemical causes, available treatments and prognosis.*

This book will be useful to anyone with chronic fatigue and malaise, light-headedness, passing out spells, chest pain, pounding in the chest or heart racing and other symptoms of dysautonomia or other illnesses with related manifestations.

Dr. Davies refers to MVPS by the alternate acronym MVPD (MVP Dysautonomia). More on this naming confusion in Chapter 5.

Chapter 3
My 5 Patient Principles and
How They Protect Me

Why do I need principles? When I'm sick, scared and confused, I depend on my 5 Patient Principles to help me make the best decisions possible without being compromised by fear or trauma. I turned to these principles, developed during my work as a reporter, to navigate MVPS flare-ups.

How I Developed My Principles

Based on my values, beliefs, and logic, these principles, though not perfect, have served me well in making important health choices. These personal guideposts provided a lifeline that saved me from making poor decisions.

This is what helped to lead me out of the deep, dark, MVPS abyss. Anyone can develop their own principles based on their unique values and needs.

The following are mine.

Principle 1
MVPS Symptoms Are Physical, Not Emotional

An emotional response to a physical problem is not the problem itself. In my experience, doctors often focus on the emotional (autonomic nervous system) reaction to MVPS instead of the problem itself.

I can go to the ER with chest pain and be afraid, but the chest pain, not the anxiety, led me to seek medical assistance.

Anxiety Is a Symptom

A doctor focused on the emotional reaction may diagnose a psychiatric cause, overlooking the potentially serious underlying problem.

There are medical conditions that can cause anxiety. For instance, a heart attack can cause anxiety.

In the Mayo Clinic Staff web article, "Heart Attack Symptoms: Know What's a Medical Emergency," the cardiac symptom is described in this way: "You may feel a sense of doom or feel as if you're having a panic attack for no apparent reason."

What Else Can It Be?

Even though I am not having a cardiac event, I do experience chest pain. The cause of that symptom should be the point of my physician's focus. If I arrived in the ER after a car accident, crying and shaking, imagine the potential consequences if the doctors treated the emotional reaction with antianxiety drugs instead of examining me for possible injuries?

A similar situation often happens with my MVPS symptoms. The emotional reaction gets the attention, not the problem that brought me to the doctor. Of course I'm scared and concerned about my health. Who wouldn't be with all the frightening symptoms of MVPS? Unless a symptom is found to be benign, I need to know if it's alerting me to something serious. MVPS symptoms usually feel profoundly serious and are often listed among the symptoms of conditions requiring immediate medical care.

My migraine headaches, for instance, are always auras that mimic most of the symptoms of a stroke. I can't risk assuming MVPS is the culprit and ignore my condition. A friend once asked me why I went to the ER multiple times when I had already been told that my chest pains were not serious—a question that raises another confusing characteristic of MVPS symptoms. They change.

For example, a pain that strikes in the center of my chest during one episode will shoot down my left arm and up to my left jaw the next, or manifest in the upper back.

A migraine that usually sends tingling down one side of my body will, out of the blue, block vision in one eye and cause my blood pressure to skyrocket.

A symptom previously evaluated as "not serious" can and does feel new and different even if it occurs in the same part of my body. It isn't so much where it occurs but more how it feels. I go back to the doctor or the ER because I can't be certain that what I'm experiencing is the same problem evaluated previously.

As long as tests are run to rule out life-threatening conditions, something I cannot assess myself, I don't care if a doctor treats me as if I am a hypochondriac. I will never accept a psychiatric diagnosis, nor will I let my symptoms be attributed to my emotional state.

In dealing with this confusing syndrome with all its frightening and ever-changing symptoms, it is in my best interest to find out the physiological cause of the symptoms.

Principle 2
A Symptom Is a Clue Not a Disease

In my experience, treating recurring symptoms as a chronic health issue does not usually fix the underlying problem.

Consider how many doctors address recurring ear infections in children. The physician treats the bacterial infection with antibiotics, which resolve the episode until the bacteria builds up again.

Doctors know that recurring ear infections are due to fluid in the middle ear that cannot drain down the eustachian tube. The fluid harbors bacteria. If the fluid could drain, the bacteria would not be able to grow and cause an infection.

Sometimes doctors recommend surgery to insert tubes in the ear to facilitate drainage, which can permanently damage the eardrum

Even the repeated use of antibiotics can cause allergies and reactions or contribute to the larger problem of creating "superbugs" the drugs can no longer kill.

There are, however, noninvasive ways to help the ears drain naturally. The infection is a symptom of the underlying problem—improper fluid drainage.

The same can be said about MVPS. If a doctor wants to treat me for anxiety because I present appearing nervous and shaking, he or she will miss the problem. The symptoms are a result of the release of adrenaline which can be due to MVPS or even some other very serious medical conditions. A doctor willing to see the symptom as a clue can probe deeper to find the real cause of the patient's discomfort.

However, identifying the symptom with a "name" can direct treatment away from the cause by focusing only on the symptom. Then prescribing a drug to cover that symptom can make a health problem worse, something I have faced many times when offered a new drug to address one of my MVPS symptoms.

Treating My IBS Symptom

Understand that symptom relief is not always a bad thing. Most everyone—myself included—has taken an over-the-counter pain reliever for a headache. I have also taken prescription medications, especially for my irritable bowel syndrome (IBS).

Painful stomach cramps have caused me to vomit and almost pass out. Fortunately, I found an old, established and effective medication I take at the onset of those cramps. The drug works fast and reduces or stops the pain entirely.

The drug does not treat the cause of IBS, although some doctors with whom I have consulted have recommended daily use as a preventative treatment. I choose to take the medication only when needed to avoid side effects. Continuous use could also render the medication ineffective.

But I am grateful to have it and take it to manage my IBS pain while I continue to look for treatments that will address the underlying problem.

Be Careful!

My gastroenterologist offered me a new, highly publicized drug touted as a breakthrough treatment for IBS. I declined. Not long after that offer, the medication was recalled after having been found to cause severe gastrointestinal complications, including ischemic colitis (a restriction in blood supply to tissues), severe constipation, hospitalizations and death.

Much has been written about the dangers of new drugs. A good introduction to this issue by Sydney Lupkin can be found on the National Public Radio website: "One-Third Of New Drugs Had Safety Problems After FDA Approval" (9 May 2017).

Before and After the MVPS Diagnosis

At the point at which my cardiac symptoms sent me to the ER three times in one month, I made an appointment with a new cardiologist to look for ways to identify or stop the chest pains.

He gave me a blank look when I said I had mitral valve prolapse syndrome. During the remainder of our conversation he would not acknowledge MVPS as a physical diagnosis, insisting instead that job-related stress caused my chest pains. Because I worked as an administrator in the hospital where he taught and practiced, he accorded me some respect, but still offered no helpful solutions or treatment.

Several months later, I went back for a follow-up. Despite his prior attitude, I needed to see him a final time to recheck a previous false-positive EKG.

On this visit, I saw the same person but found a completely different physician—one who had just returned from a conference, which included a lecture on MVPS. He put his hand on my shoulder and said, "I know how difficult this MVPS has been for you, and I have learned some things that might help."

Really, what? Something new? Something helpful?

No. He offered me drugs with some scary side effects to cover the symptoms.

What did my cardiologist actually learn at the conference? He learned exactly what the drug company wanted him to know. They taught him how to diagnose and treat MVPS with one or more of the drugs they manufactured. In my experience, the practice of medicine today involves arriving at a diagnosis for which a drug exists to cover the symptoms.

I declined the doctor's offer of a prescription, coming away from the encounter with the cold comfort that people like me were finally being validated as having MVPS—but only because that validation supported a drug company's marketing strategy.

Thanks, Big Pharma.

But a Diagnosis Will Not Cure Me

For more than thirty years I have lived with my MVPS diagnosis but naming the condition has not led to a cure. Looking beyond the diagnosis can, however, reveal underlying issues.

For example, I have also been diagnosed with benign arrhythmias, a common symptom of MVPS. The calcium channel blockers routinely used to treat arrhythmia, however, carry serious side effects.

Another doctor looked deeper, tested my magnesium level and found it to be low—a proven cause of arrhythmias.

I was given magnesium to bring my levels back to normal, which stopped the arrhythmias.

I continue to take magnesium to maintain my levels.

I rarely read about any side effects other than loose bowels. It is commonly used to gently treat constipation when taken as Milk of Magnesia. However, some people with kidney problems or other health issues may not be candidates for this mineral.

Readers can find a thorough discussion of magnesium's role as a natural calcium channel blocker in Dr. Mark Houston's article:

"The Role of Magnesium in Hypertension and Cardiovascular Disease," which appeared in the 26 September 2011 issue of *The Journal of Clinical Hypertension.*

So long as I remember that a symptom is not a disease, I seem to get better care and find more options. Sometimes I need symptom relief and will accept treatment, but I do not fool myself into thinking that intervention addresses the actual problem.

When a doctor begins to discuss psychiatric sources for my symptoms, I know I've reached a dead-end street where I will never find answers to my health issues because I know that my MVPS symptoms are physical, not emotional.

Principle 3
Be Sure Tests and Treatments are Necessary and Not Worse Than the Problem

Before I agree to a treatment or test, I want to be fully informed about potential risks so that I may weigh those factors against possible benefits. Treatments and tests can cause permanent damage or even death.

Tests Carry Risks Too

For the most part, I am reasonably comfortable with tests that include urine, blood, stool and any other noninvasive assessments. Those tests that include cutting, injecting or inserting instruments into the body give me pause. This includes X-rays where radiation penetrates the tissue.

According to the unsigned article,

"Understanding Radiation Risk from Imaging Tests," which appears on The American Cancer Society web page, radiation exposure from all sources can add up over a lifetime and increase the risk of cancer.

CTs vs. MRIs

When a lump appeared on the front of my neck, an ear, nose, and throat specialist (ENT) to whom I was referred decided the mass had no relation to the benign cysts that have appeared for years on my thyroid. Since I could see the large lump in the mirror, I was understandably concerned with the doctor's evaluation.

A Computerized Tomography Scan (CT)

The ENT ordered a computerized tomography (CT) scan of my thyroid. The procedure takes a series of X-ray images from different angles. I asked if a magnetic resonance imaging (MRI) scan would provide the same information. The doctor told me the MRI would actually provide superior information and was safer. Radiation exposure makes the thyroid vulnerable to the development of cancer. I opted for the MRI.

*(*For more information on the link between radiation and thyroid cancer, see the unsigned article, "By the way, doctor: How does radiation cause thyroid cancer?" Harvard Women's Health Watch, February 2007.*)*

The doctor admitted that he originally offered the CT scan because most people don't like to be in the tightly enclosed area required by the MRI. I am still amazed that he didn't present both options and allow me to make the choice.

After more probing and drawing from my own experiences with both tests, I felt that the MRI provided the best option, was medically necessary and did not present a larger danger than the problem itself.

An MRI

Unlike CT scans or X-rays, an MRI does not use ionizing radiation that may cause DNA damage or cancer. However, injected gadolinium contrast that can be used to enhance the MRI image sometimes lingers in the body and can change or damage the brain when used six or more times.

(See: Guo, Bang J., Zhen L. Yang, and Long J. Zhang, "Gadolinium Deposition in Brain: Current Scientific Evidence and Future Perspectives," Frontiers in Molecular Neuroscience, 2018: 11.)

At the imaging center, I learned the doctor had ordered an MRI with contrast. He had not discussed that with me. I declined the contrast even after assurances from the staff that adverse reactions are rare. Don't care.

I signed a waiver and did the MRI without contrast, which, as it turned out, provided all the information needed. My doctor was wrong. The lump was not in my throat but, instead, was a benign cyst on my thyroid gland and treatable with a medication adjustment.

Two factors influenced my decision. First, I want to save MRIs with contrast for something more serious if ever needed. Second, an MRI without contrast can be revealing in its own right and has no known side effects.

(For more information on MRIs, see "Magnetic Resonance Imaging [MRI Scan]" by William C. Shiel Jr., MD, FACP, FACR on MedicineNet.")

Finally, I canceled my follow-up appointment with the ENT. If a doctor, especially one in his specialty, couldn't tell the difference between my throat and my thyroid, then I knew I needed to find a new physician.

Treatment Risks

In the United States, drugs are the most common treatment options, an approach I find problematic on many levels. Too many times when I look at the risks of specific drugs, the potential side effects are worse than the problem itself.

For example, many cardiac drugs can cause heart attacks. What if I had taken the deadly IBS drug that was pulled from the market and had suffered one of the side effects? IBS, although extremely painful, will not kill me. The drug that was recommended to me as a "cure" might, however, prove lethal.

In addition to drug sensitivities, I have problems recovering from medical procedures. This fact leads me to pick and choose interventions with the most benefit and the least harm. Sometimes a treatment isn't even needed as most of my MVPS symptoms come and go anyway.

There are many reasons to pause and think before accepting any medical advice. Consider the press release "Study Suggests Medical Errors Now Third Leading Cause of Death in the U.S.: Physicians advocate for changes in how deaths are reported to better reflect reality," released by Johns Hopkins on 3 May 2016.

The release discusses a study, which determined that more than 250,000 U.S. citizens die annually due to medical mistakes, making such errors the third leading cause of death after heart disease and cancer at the time of publication.

The study was also discussed in an article by Ray Sipherd for CNBC, "The Third-Leading Cause of Death in US Most Doctors Don't Want You to Know About," 22 February 2018.

I research any drug prescribed to me before taking it and often speak with my pharmacists about the medication.

After reading in various reports that doctors are ill-informed about the side-effects of the drugs they prescribe, I have made questioning prescriptions a matter of habit.

(See: Jonathan Weiss, "Doctors Don't Know The Side Effects Of The Drugs They Prescribe; Pharma Reps To Blame," *Medical Daily*, 29 May 2013.

Amanda Gardner, "Doctors Not Heeding 'Black-Box' Warnings on Rx Drugs," *HealthDay*, 18 November 2005.

Lauran Neergaard, "FDA Cast Doubts on Doctors" ABC News, January 6, 2006

Risks: Probability vs. Possibility

Only I can weigh the risks and benefits when I am the one who will have to deal with the consequences. If death or a nonreversible side effect is the risk and my life is not on the line, I look for other options. A doctor may tell me that the risk is low, but if I happen to be one of the people who suffer a particular side effect, the "low" risk turns out to be 100% for me.

The Risk of No Treatment:

The Case for Antibiotic Prophylaxis (Preventive Treatment)

At diagnosis, the only treatment my cardiologist recommended for my MVPS was an antibiotic protocol before surgery or dental procedures to prevent endocarditis, an infection of the inner lining of the heart chambers and heart valves.

The serious, potentially life-threatening infection occurs when germs from another part of the body, such as the mouth, spread through the bloodstream and attach themselves to damaged areas in the heart.

After fifteen years of adhering to this advice, during which I took antibiotics before dental work and medical procedures, the recommendation for mild MVPS sufferers changed. Preventive antibiotics were no longer considered necessary. I read the report detailing the basis for the recommendation and decided to continue my personal use of preventative antibiotics. I don't take antibiotics often, nor do I have adverse reactions to them. The reputed "risk" of taking antibiotics did not seem to apply to me.

An updated report on this recommendation was released by the American Heart Association in 2019 as presented on the American Dental Association website.

The text reads in part, "Infective endocarditis prophylaxis for dental procedures should be recommended only for patients with underlying cardiac conditions associated with the highest risk of adverse outcome from infective endocarditis."

(See the unsigned article, "Antibiotic Prophylaxis Prior to Dental Procedures," *American Dental Association.*)

The recommendation is based on the low odds of mild MVPS sufferers contracting endocarditis. I prefer to err on the side of caution.

What are the odds that I will be one of the unlucky "few" people who do end up with endocarditis?

According to an article by Grace Rattue, "Patients With Infective Endocarditis And Heart Failure Have Reduced Mortality With Valvular Surgery," *Medical News Today*, 24 November 2011:

"Infective endocarditis is associated with substantial morbidity and mortality. Several published studies have reported in-hospital mortality of 15 percent to 20 percent and 1-year mortality of 40 percent. In the United States alone, approximately 15,000 new cases of infective endocarditis are diagnosed each year."

My decision to accept or reject a treatment will always be based on the associated risks, not the calculated odds of something occurring. For me, the risk of endocarditis outweighs the risk of taking antibiotics. So the question I ask myself is whether I want to take the risk of the side effect, not whether I want to play the odds with my health. I always weigh the risk. The decision to take a medication is not a Las Vegas game of chance. I don't play the odds when it comes to my life. I rely on one sure guideline: be sure tests and treatments are not worse than the problem itself.

The reverse can also be true. Refusing a treatment may hold more risk than taking the drug. I weigh each option for potential benefits and choose the treatment that offers the best outcome with the least potential harm.

Principle 4
One Protocol Does Not Work for Everyone

Doctors usually offer a diagnosis and treatment based on accepted guidelines for the practice of medicine. Insurance companies, hospital departments, state medical boards and other professional and regulating organizations develop those protocols.

Such guidelines aim to assist physicians with decision-making to maintain consistent and high medical standards. My personal concern, however, is the risk of a doctor falling back on a preconceived medical practice before conducting a complete evaluation of my situation.

My unique health issues are not well understood or commonly treated by conventional medicine. I am a square peg that does not fit conventional medicine's round hole—no matter how hard they try to hammer me in place.

In the hospital I am almost always subjected to guidelines referred to as "standard of care" or "standing orders." Such approaches may be a good rule of thumb or a viable starting point for a more thorough evaluation, but if I were to allow physicians to force me to fit their preconceived standards, my condition could be made worse.

Apparently I am not the only one who sees this as a problem. Steven H. Woolf, professor of family medicine, and Jeremy Grimshaw, professor of public health, published in *The BMJ* (the medical journal of the British Medical Association) in February 1999, discuss "Potential Benefits, Limitations, and Harms of Clinical Guidelines."

The authors determine that the benefits of clinical guidelines are not clear "due to the fact that patients, doctors, payers, and managers define quality differently and because current evidence about the effectiveness of guidelines is incomplete."

My Experience with Standing Orders

In a single hospital visit, I had two experiences with "standing orders." Neither was useful. The first occurred during an ER intake, and the second was during the hospital stay.

According to the definition provided in *Mosby's Medical Dictionary, 9th edition. © 2009, Elsevier*, standing orders in a hospital setting usually name the condition and prescribe the action to be taken. The order includes instructions for the administration of treatments and when to give a drug or perform a therapeutic procedure.

On my first experience, I went to the ER with right-side weakness of the body and loss of sight in the right eye. My blood pressure, usually around 110/70 spiked to 170/83 and did not respond to medication. I was afraid that I might be having a stroke.

A friend took me to the ER. The first triage question the nurse asked when I described my symptoms was whether or not I'd had a flu shot. I was stunned. What did a vaccination have to do with a potential stroke?

Ultimately I learned that administering vaccines falls within the standard of care for all patients. Since antibodies do not develop for two weeks after a flu shot has been received, the vaccine question did not address my safety or theirs.

In my opinion, had the medical professionals wanted to ask about the status of my flu shot, they should have waited until the emergency for which I sought help had been resolved.

The nurse questioned my assertion that I have serious reactions to vaccines as my records indicated. I politely reminded her that I had come to the ER seeking an evaluation for stroke-like symptoms.

Patients are told to get to a hospital within the "golden hour" following the onset of such symptoms.

As the axiom goes, "time lost is brain lost." Clot-busting drugs must be administered within that window to prevent permanent damage.

I would have thought that potential stroke symptoms, not the question of whether I had received a flu shot, would have been the priority.

However, the hospital's standard of care required the nurse to discuss flu shots with me during that critical window of treatment opportunity.

Because my EKG appeared somewhat outside the norm, I remained under observation in the hospital for twenty-three hours. In the end, however, it was determined that I had experienced a migraine headache that presented with what were for me new neurological symptoms.

I remained stable during that entire time. When the hospital doctor came to my room to discharge me, he claimed that he had been following my case all night and held my file to confirm that level of attention. I had never seen him before.

During our conversation, he directed me to follow up with my cardiologist but recommended that I take the blood thinner Plavix even though my blood was not thick or clotting. He also recommended a cholesterol-reducing statin regardless of levels that registered normal for my age.

Finally, he suggested a beta blocker for cardiac symptoms, which every doctor with whom I had consulted previously assured me was not necessary for my problems. At the end of our conversation, the hospital doctor handed me the necessary prescriptions. Later that same week, I saw my personal doctor who did not recommend the three-drug regimen.

That was more than seven years ago. I have been fine without the drugs. To me, that ER visit offers a perfect example of standing orders that did not reflect my healthcare needs.

I am always careful that I am not being placed into a standard medical protocol where I do not belong. I know from experience how this can cause more problems for me instead of providing the help I need. One protocol does not work for everyone.

Principle 5
Trust Myself

No one knows my medical history and symptoms, or how my body works, acts, and reacts better than I do. No one else has been there with me 24/7. I am the only expert on me.

No one can give me the right answer for my healthcare without respecting my input. I listen, research (if there is time), and learn. I am open to information and advice. My goal is to access any key information that helps me to decide if an option offered fits my circumstances, feels right and makes sense.

The Best Doctors Listen to Their Patients

Sir William Osler, a nineteenth-century Canadian physician and one of the four founding professors of Johns Hopkins Hospital, knew that doctors who listen to their patients have the most direct path to finding the problem. Osler said, "Listen to your patient; he is telling you the diagnosis."

If I hold the answer, I have an even greater responsibility to listen to my body. Even in the confusion of MVPS, I know what I am currently feeling, how I have felt in the past, and what symptoms I have. I need a doctor who will take the time to listen to me as the best means to arrive at an accurate diagnosis.

Combining what I know about my body and what the doctor knows about medicine can and should be a powerful collaboration.

Listen to That Little Voice

We've all heard about the wise little voice that whispers the truth only to be ignored or shouted down by outside pressures or influences. I try to listen to that voice—especially when my health is on the line. In hindsight, that voice has almost never been wrong.

Whether that voice is a gut feeling, an intuition, or an instinct, I recognize the feeling of unease before a treatment or when a doctor asks a question that doesn't quite make sense.

Eric Haseltine, Ph.D., discusses this inner wisdom in his *Psychology Today* article, "Yes, You Have a Sixth Sense, and You Should Trust It," (25 April 2015). Haseltine writes, "...there are scientifically valid reasons to *trust* your feelings, perceptions, and intuitions, even when you can't sense how you sense them."

I have learned to respect my self-knowledge and to listen to that nagging voice begging to be heard. When in doubt, I do nothing until I figure out my situation and options.

If the answers are in me, I need to listen to and trust myself. In truth, no one can tell me what I need, want or believe. I have to find those answers for myself even when I need help doing it.

Refusing to discount myself ranks in equal importance to finding a doctor who will not discount me.

Chapter 4
Five Conflicting Characteristics of the MVPS Diagnosis and How Knowing Them Has Helped My Treatment

Over the years I have adjusted to the ever-changing names for my condition. I have been told I have mitral valve prolapse (MVP), mitral valve prolapse syndrome (MVPS), MVPS-Dysautonomia (MVPS-D), and MVP dysautonomia (MVPD). The medical tests have also changed during that time for both diagnosing and refuting the condition.

Mitral Valve Prolapse Diagnosis

On initial diagnosis of mitral valve prolapse (MVP), the doctor described this "click-murmur syndrome" as an instance in which overly large valve leaflets fail to close smoothly, making a clicking sound. Other names for the harmless condition included Barlow's syndrome and floppy valve syndrome.

Some people with MVP require treatment when the valve does not close completely and causes regurgitation. The blood leaks back through the valve instead of moving forward. This real, visible pathological and physical problem can be serious enough to require surgery.

Fortunately, I do not have regurgitation, mitral valve issues, or any cardiac problems. My collection of symptoms has been referred to as mitral valve prolapse syndrome - dysautonomia.

The MVP and the MVPS Disconnect

At diagnosis I was assured I had a functioning, healthy heart with a valve that closed completely. With that good news, I went back to my life. Nothing had changed except the presence of a click as the mitral valve closed, noted by some doctors during physical exams, and occasional mild flutters. MVP symptoms like palpitations, shortness of breath, cough, fatigue, dizziness, anxiety, migraine headaches and chest discomfort can come and go or disappear for years.

For more information, you can read the unsigned article "Mitral Valve Prolapse" on the National Heart, Lung, and Blood Institute's webpage.

Looking back, I experienced mild and intermittent instances of some of those symptoms long before I was diagnosed. At first, I never found those issues problematic, and I failed to connect any of them to MVP. Many years later, everything changed, beginning with stroke-like weakness down one side of my body. Chest pain became a recurring symptom, followed by daily arrhythmias, irritable bowel episodes and a litany of other classic MVPS symptoms.

The MVPS Diagnosis
Characteristic-1
A Floppy Valve with Unrelated Symptoms

When my mitral valve prolapse problems began, I didn't know what was happening. As the symptoms mounted, I feared I would die, and I felt that no one was helping me. That was when I turned to the internet.

I can still remember sitting in my chair in the dead of night wrapped in a blanket with a cup of hot tea, glued to the monitor. My fears escalated as I searched my symptoms and read the serious conditions that were associated with them. Then an MVPS website popped up that gave me pause. I was told I had MVP. What was the "syndrome"?

After visiting multiple websites, I leaned back with tears of relief filling my eyes. I had MVPS. Several more doctors would come and go before a medical professional confirmed my diagnosis, but I knew I was right. Finding a benign reason for my symptoms gave me my life back—I was okay.

Or Was I?

With time, I began to doubt that my problems could be explained by a benign syndrome. It became harder to attribute the constellation of worsening and multiplying issues to MVPS. When symptoms flared, I experienced a cascading event. One issue led to another until I found myself in a full-blown episode of an MVPS flare-up. I felt no relief knowing that I only had MVPS.

Is Everything MVPS?

The frightening arrhythmias and chest pains could easily have been caused by a separate issue. As I grew older, I could not ignore the fact that women in high-stress jobs often suffered heart attacks in their forties.

Who was to say that a person with MVPS could not have a heart attack or throw a clot when all my symptoms could be interpreted as warnings of just such an event? Additionally, I had a ton of frightening noncardiac symptoms that were, at times, debilitating. A stomach bleed, for instance, put me in the hospital for two days.

The MVPS Symptoms

My list of symptoms kept growing, but from what I have read, each individual experiences a unique combination of what can seem to be an unlimited list of MVPS-related problems.

A minor symptom for me could cause someone else greater issues. The following list represents the typical MVPS symptoms. I have experienced those marked with an asterisk and will not be surprised if I face more in the future.

- Chest pain*

- Palpitations or irregular heartbeat (arrhythmias)*

- Migraine headaches with pain

- Migraine auras with stroke-like symptoms*

- Difficulty with balance

- Fainting or near-fainting spells

- Shortness of breath*

- Shakiness*

- Cold sweats/weak feeling*

- Dizziness/vertigo*

- Numbness in any part of the body*

- Trouble with eyes or visual disturbances*

- Fatigue*

- Hypersensitivities/easily startled*

- Sleep problems*

- Anxiety*

- Depression

- Panic attacks with pounding heartbeat*

- Irritable bowel syndrome*

- Gastroesophageal reflux disease (GERD)*

- Sensitivity to drugs, caffeine, and medications*

- Allergies*

- Asthma/bronchitis

- Aches or pains*

- Back problems*

- Bladder problems*

- Skin irritations and rashes*

- Muscle fatigue or weakness*

- Muscular tensions/twitching*

- Difficulty concentrating*

- Chemical sensitivities and food allergies*

The realization that my MVP had morphed into MVPS changed my view of the problem and its treatment. I couldn't count on my past knowledge.

Any of the first ten symptoms listed above would, for the general population, signal a serious health problem or even a medical emergency—but not for me. These symptoms can be my daily fare.

When a symptom flares, I often have to remind myself that I am not in danger and act according to the plan I've developed. The plan is specific for each issue, which helps me treat the problem more effectively as well as determine its risk.

The MVPS Diagnosis
Characteristic-2
MVPS Looks Like Other Syndromes

The deeper I searched the MVPS diagnosis, the more I discovered symptoms that overlapped with other disorders. My symptoms also appeared among those for fibromyalgia and chronic fatigue syndrome.

I refer to both conditions as MVPS "sister syndromes." My research indicated that people who did not carry my diagnosis also suffered from many of my symptoms. Why was that the case? Could researching those disorders lead me to answers for my issues? There was only one way to find out.

A Look at Fibromyalgia

Fibromyalgia and chronic fatigue syndrome summaries emphasize symptoms that best represent the particular diagnosis. For example, fibromyalgia information predominately addresses widespread muscle and tissue pain.

I experience flare-ups of both. My skin can become exquisitely painful to the barest touch. That discomfort, however, does not figure heavily among MVPS symptoms nor even as an aspect of my personal list of symptoms.

My MVPS list usually starts with cardiac symptoms such as racing or irregular heartbeat (arrhythmia), chest pain and shortness of breath. All are associated with fibromyalgia and chronic fatigue syndrome, but not prominently.

Reports note that many people with fibromyalgia describe intense, sharp, or stabbing pain in the chest and ribs, which tends to be attributed to costochondritis, an inflammation of the rib cage.

Again, I have been diagnosed with costochondritis and cannot touch some areas of my ribs when they are inflamed. This particular symptom of pain has confused my diagnosis with gallbladder dysfunction, which presents at the tip of the right, lower rib. More often than not, however, the types of chest pains that send me to the ER are esophageal spasms that eerily mimic a heart attack.

I found familiar symptoms among those listed for fibromyalgia, including migraine headaches and irritable bowel syndrome—and, interestingly, mitral valve prolapse.

That's right. Some people with fibromyalgia could also have MVP as a symptom.

I came away feeling as if someone dumped all the word tiles from one board game and reorganized them to fit the rules of another. People with fibromyalgia appeared to have all the same symptoms that plagued me but presented in a different order of emphasis.

Research supports the inclusion of MVP as a symptom of fibromyalgia. In "Prevalence of Mitral Valve Prolapse in Primary Fibromyalgia: A Pilot Investigation," published in the July 1989 edition of *Archives of Physical Medicine and Rehabilitation*, authors M.J. Pellegrino, D. Van Fossen, C. Gordon, J.M. Ryan and G.W. Waylonis, theorized that MVP may be part of a more generalized connective tissue abnormality.

Really? My research on MVPS did not include that reasoning. The information I encountered most often purported that the prolapse is hereditary and a marker for dysautonomia.

I had no reason to doubt that characterization. My mother suffered from almost all the symptoms listed as MVPS back in the 1960s although she was never diagnosed.

Both she and her mother often complained of cardiac symptoms with no underlying pathology. I might add that both were considered hypochondriacs. In my experience, doctors tend to fall back on that stereotype when they don't understand or have not studied the problems that are presented to them.

I have also found that some MVPS symptoms can be listed as symptoms of another MVPS symptom. For example, IBS can be noted as a primary medical problem with a list of associated problems.

One study I read showed that people with IBS are more likely to have other disorders, including migraines, fibromyalgia, and depression. (J. Alexander Cole, Kenneth J. Rothma, et al, "Migraine, Fibromyalgia, and Depression Among People with IBS: A Prevalence Study," *BMC Gastroenterology*, June 2006.)

This information offers an excellent example of the intertwined nature of symptoms.

I am personally irritated that anxiety and depression seem to be gratuitously added to such symptom lists. In my experience, adding those psychiatric disorders often prevents doctors from focusing on the main problems at hand.

A Closer Look at the Anxiety and Depression Diagnosis

In my opinion, psychiatry has become too intricately involved in the diagnostic process whether needed or not. I believe that fluctuating human emotions are mostly natural, not psychiatric.

Anxiety

Anxiety can consist of numerous symptoms: an impending sense of doom or danger, accelerated heart rate, rapid breathing, sweating, shaking, a feeling of weakness, nervousness, and panic.

Physiologically, the hormone adrenaline causes anxiety and fear. Gratuitous adrenaline release underlies dysautonomia, which causes the majority of MVPS symptoms.

To my thinking, physiological reactions to adrenaline release is a common feature of MVPS, not a psychiatric problem of anxiety.

Though commonly excreted during times of stress and fear, adrenaline release is not necessarily caused by emotional factors or tied to a psychiatric disorder.

In many instances, adrenaline prepares the body to react to danger and trauma in a lifesaving way. The hormone can temporarily block the pain from serious injury and restrict blood vessels to lessen life-threatening bleeding until medical attention can be sought.

People suffering from heart attacks experience anxiety. The same adrenaline that causes that feeling can, under different circumstances, help a heart to continue to beat.

For more information on these characteristics of adrenaline, see: "What is Adrenaline?" *Hormone Health Network*

"Heart Attack Symptoms: Know What's a Medical Emergency," Mayo Clinic.

"Adrenaline Can Restart the Heart but is No Good for the Brain," 4 September 2018, National Institute for Health Research.

Not Always a Good Thing

I can calmly watch a happy movie on television when an unexpected adrenaline surge triggers anxiety and fear followed by one or more MVPS symptoms. This happens in the absence of upset, fear, nervousness, or worry.

The incident cannot be traced to childhood memories or PTSD. No amount of therapy will stop such episodes, and an anxiety diagnosis followed by drug treatment will not find or address the unprovoked physiological event.

In a stressful situation, the extra adrenaline in my body can turn nervousness into anxiety which then can trigger a panic attack. Now that I understand that sequence, I no longer overreact, which helps calm everything down. More on this in Chapter 16: Breakthrough Treatments That Changed My Life.

Depression

Even though I have had IBS, migraines, and fibromyalgia symptoms, I resent depression being casually dropped into the mix. That inclusion discounts everything else I've experienced.

Depression can be caused by underlying health and physiological issues. (See: Mary Ann Block, *Just Because You're Depressed Doesn't Mean You Have Depression*, 28 April 2008.)

From my point of view and experience, when high levels of adrenaline run through my body causing anxiety and a host of MVPS symptoms, I don't feel happy. During those times, if I feel down, blue or depressed, it is with good reason.

A diagnosis of depression paired with a prescription for an antidepressant won't fix the cause of that feeling. Anyone living with the list of symptoms for fibromyalgia and MVPS has ample and normal reasons to feel down or depressed, especially during flare-ups.

Are the majority of people attending a funeral suffering from the symptoms of depression, or are they just naturally sad? Should everyone who experiences deep sadness take an antidepressant?

I would prefer to experience this normal reaction to loss by relying on the natural process to grieve and then heal.

To me, adding an inaccurate psychiatric diagnosis of depression to my list of symptoms can allow a doctor to simply suggest

I take an antidepressant—a class of drugs that carry significant risks and side effects. I prefer my doctors to help with the chronic MVPS symptoms that can sometimes cause me to feel depressed rather than simply prescribing a drug to mask the symptom of depression.

In my frame of reference, depression is natural. I may need to grieve for what I have lost in order to accept the loss, start over, and move forward. That philosophy has always worked for me.

Common Symptoms of Fibromyalgia

Those items bearing an asterisk are symptoms I experience with MVPS. The overlap of symptoms between fibromyalgia and MVPS is obvious.

• Pain and tender points*

- Fatigue*

- Sleep problems*

- Concentration and memory problems, known as "fibro fog" *

- Anxiety*

- Depression

- Morning stiffness*

- Numbness and tingling in hands, arms, feet, and legs*

- Headaches*

- Irritable bowel syndrome*

- Urinary problems*

- Sensitivity to cold or heat*

- Dizziness*

- Chest symptoms*

- Breathing problems*

Chronic Fatigue Syndrome, The Other Sister Syndrome

My personal research revealed articles and documentaries exposing the unfairness of the benign name "chronic fatigue syndrome," and suggested what amounts to a conspiracy by medical professionals to discount the seriousness of the condition.

Only recently has chronic fatigue syndrome (CFS) been recognized as a real and serious problem, which is now also referred to as myalgic encephalomyelitis (ME). Accepted as more accurate to the underlying issue, the new name is not descriptive, however, of the more profound yet often discounted symptom of fatigue.

That doctors do not question the fatigue that often occurs with other health issues amazes me. Unrelenting fatigue can be indicative of some chronic underlying problem. (See: The Mayo Clinic staff article, "Symptoms: Fatigue")

"Myalgic" means related to the nerves or nerve pain. "Encephalomyelitis" refers to inflammation of the brain and spinal cord, typically due to acute viral infection. Taken singularly or in combination, these words do not refer to little things.

To learn more, see the *New York Times* opinion piece (18 March 2017) by Julie Rehmeyer and David Tuller, "Getting It Wrong on Chronic Fatigue Syndrome."

Those still living with this syndrome may derive some comfort from being validated after suffering the long-term perception that they are somehow malingering. That validation does not, however, relieve their symptoms or daily pain.

People with CFS/ME experience overwhelming fatigue that sleep or rest does not alleviate. They lack the energy for simple, everyday tasks like preparing a meal, showering, or dressing.

Anyone who has ever been knocked down by the flu can understand the feeling of being unable to function, but unlike the flu, CFS/ME fatigue does not resolve in a few days. Some CFS/ME sufferers become completely disabled.

Some of the more common symptoms in addition to the fatigue of CFS/ME include:

- Muscle and joint pain and aches
- Headaches
- Flu-like symptoms

- Digestive issues, like irritable bowel syndrome
- Chills and night sweats
- Allergies and sensitivities to foods, odors, chemicals, or noise

I have had all of these symptoms, but the occasional fatigue I feel is not as severe as those diagnosed with CFS/ME.

Other Markers for CFS/ME

I also have been tested and shown positive for the Epstein-Barr virus (EBV) and Lyme disease, both associated with CFS but not commonly connected to MVPS.

Epstein-Barr can cause mononucleosis or "mono," and although it can resolve in a few weeks, EBV can sometimes become chronic. Initial symptoms include fatigue, headaches, fever, sore throat and swollen lymph nodes. In some cases, chronic fatigue and swollen glands and a general feeling of being unwell can persist for months to years.

Lyme disease is caused by a type of bacteria carried by deer ticks. An infected tick can transmit the bacteria through its bite. If treated early, the disease can be cured with antibiotics. Cases that go undetected can cause chronic symptoms involving the joints, heart, and nervous system.

(See: "Symptoms of Post-Treatment Lyme Disease Syndrome," Healthline.)

Is CFS/ME the manifestation of EBV and Lyme disease, or does CFS/ME represent a complicating factor in an already confusing diagnosis? Either way, in my estimation, they each need to be treated.

The Underlying Condition

Comparing the similarities between MVPS, fibromyalgia, or CFS/ME reveals many overlapping symptoms. The distinction in names does not alter the fact that sufferers experience differing degrees of the same symptoms.

What if an underlying condition exists that causes these similarities in MVPS, fibromyalgia and CFS/ME? Could that common denominator cause the overlapping symptoms?

The MVPS Diagnosis
Characteristic-3
A Syndrome Is Not a Disease

The MVPS diagnosis helped me to research and learns more about this life-altering health problem and reassured me that I was not alone and dying. But I had to break out of the MVPS diagnosis to find better answers for one simple reason: MVPS is not a disease but a *syndrome*.

By definition, a "syndrome" lumps multiple unidentified symptoms together to form less of a diagnosis and more of a characterization. Inherently, this indicates no single cause or defined cure.

(See: "What Exactly Are Syndromes?" *Health:* The University of Utah.)

Disease vs. Syndrome

A disease, on the other hand, can be defined as a medical condition of the body that usually can be measured. High blood pressure would be a good example, unlike a headache which is a symptom that cannot be objectively quantified.

Symptoms are subjective. They are felt by the patient but can't be seen. That is the case for all my MVPS symptoms. Even though I can feel them, no test can find the problem. It has been my experience that some doctors who cannot see the problem tend to discount the issue and label it a wastebasket diagnosis.

See: "Sign vs. Symptom," *Medical News Today*.

A "Wastebasket" Diagnosis

According to The Free Dictionary, when a syndrome is referred to as a "garbage can" or "wastebasket" diagnosis, the inference is that the identification is not based on physiological proof and cannot be specifically described. Therefore, the thinking goes that the description is scientifically useless because it is too broadly inclusive.

I have heard the term used during my tenure working in the healthcare system. In my opinion, a wastebasket diagnosis can sometimes lead a doctor to assume an emotional root cause for a physical illness. I believe this to be evident when a patient receives a psychiatric diagnosis along with a syndrome, such as depression or anxiety commonly associated with

MVPS. Both chronic fatigue syndrome and fibromyalgia have been tagged as "wastebasket disorders."

A report that focused on myalgic encephalomyelitis/chronic fatigue syndrome (ME/CFS), published in the *Health Care Women International*, *"Dismissing chronic illness: A qualitative analysis of negative healthcare experiences,"* supports my premise.

The report states: "Our findings of this patient-focused study echo those of prior physician-focused researchers. Many participants reported being told their ME/CFS symptoms were the consequences of a psychological issue, with depression being the most frequent inappropriate attributed cause" supports my premise. In comparison to other chronic problems, little information appears online about MVPS. However, most of my symptoms are listed as a wastebasket diagnosis. These include irritable bowel syndrome, interstitial cystitis, costochondritis and gastroesophageal reflux.

To make the situation worse, many doctors I have known believe that other healthcare professionals who tried to help me with my "syndrome" were "quacks." Because those doctors had nothing to offer me, they seemed to believe that no other physicians could have answers and were therefore worthy of criticism for trying.

One doctor I consulted was adamant that I should not go on the Candida diet that one of my more helpful physicians recommended to treat my chronic yeast infections. The diet reduces foods that cause fungus growth, including gluten, sugar, alcohol products, and some dairy products but includes protein, healthful fats, vegetables, and probiotics.

The objecting doctor told me he didn't want me to waste my time on an unproven treatment. How thoughtful. He didn't change my mind, and as it turns out, the diet helped. Perhaps the actual time I wasted was spent in his office.

Selling a Syndrome

Validation of a syndrome seems to carry greater benefit for drug companies than for patients like me. Once named, a syndrome can become the focus of numerous drugs recommended for symptom control.

But I cannot stress often enough that, to me, a symptom is only a clue, not a disease. Remember that it was only after a drug company validated MVPS that a cardiologist who had previously discounted my condition changed his mind and attempted to give me a drug to ease my symptoms.

No thanks.

Drug companies referred to as "malady" or "disease" mongers are not above making up findings to increase sales, a problem discussed by John LaMattina in his *Forbes* article, "There Go Those Drug Companies Inventing New Diseases Again."

I have found no reports that any scientist has ever discovered the origin of MVPS along with an effective treatment. This leads me to wonder if some creative people working at a drug company made up a new condition by adding an "S" to the MVP diagnosis and then offered a boatload of drugs to treat the condition.

How did MVP become MVPS? I have not found an answer to that question. For that matter, how did I end up with MVP in the first place? Some doctors hear the click; others don't. Some echocardiograms have shown the valve flopping, but the two most recent ones did not.

If these negative findings are correct and I don't have MVP, then how can it be a marker for MVPS? It seems to me that I could as easily be diagnosed with either of the two sister syndromes, fibromyalgia and chronic fatigue syndrome/myalgic encephalomyelitis.

The name of the diagnosis doesn't appear to change anything for me. MVPS, fibromyalgia, and CFS/MW are all chronic conditions with no cure and similar symptoms.

I am far more interested in the underlying cause of the symptoms than the name of the condition or syndrome.

The Benefits of Letting Go of the MVP Diagnosis

Maybe I don't have MVP. My cardiologist and updated medical information have both indicated to me that the diagnosis was faulty and based on old, flawed technology that caused many false positives.

The new technology offers greater accuracy, according to my doctor. The most recent echocardiograms did not show mitral valve prolapse at all. My valve closes perfectly, and my heart is strong.

Dr. Judith Reichman from the *Today Show* reported the following in a January 2005 article:

"Improved tests, however, have led cardiologists to the conclusion that the mitral valve has normal variations and that a 'whoosh' or a 'click' does not necessarily mean a heart condition." (See: "Too Much Noise About This Heart Murmur?") So I ask again; if I don't have MVP, then how can I have MVPS?

I cannot resolve the contradictory explanation that people can have one without the other. My questions don't stop there. If the first diagnosis of MVP was false, why do physicians keep building on it? How can there ever be an effective treatment for the problem when medical science cannot explain what condition I actually have? Adding more erroneous disorders to the name does not clarify the problem for me. Why can't the medical professionals whose aid I seek change my diagnosis to reflect the actual problem?

By letting go of the name and all the treatments associated with it, my action plan became more effective—and continues to improve as I dig deeper and deeper to find the primary cause.

This is what I found. All roads lead me to the diagnosis of an instability in the autonomic nervous system. That explanation makes sense to me and addresses everything I have experienced so far and brings me light years away from that first dubious diagnosis of Mitral Valve Prolapse.

The word "dysautonomia" was added to the original MVPS diagnosis for just this reason. Though helpful, that addition did not provide answers to all my questions, but it has been a good point of focus for my action plan.

The MVPS Diagnosis
Characteristic-4
Dysautonomia

I originally thought the list of MVPS symptoms could be used as a guide to help me find my actual diagnosis. But then a new theory emerged that an instability of the autonomic nervous system (ANS), not a problem with the heart, caused my wide array of MVPS symptoms. Later statistics showed that there was a subset of patients with mitral valve prolapse who also had autonomic dysfunction and that MVP was a marker for that disorder. Patients in this group, like me, were given an updated diagnosis of "MVPS with Dysautonomia." But what if MVPS is a subset of dysautonomia? Calling my problem "MVPS-Dysautonomia" would seem to dilute the actual problem when it is the dysautonomia that should be the focus. When I mentally dropped the MVPS diagnosis, the dysautonomia did begin to make sense, but not completely.

Dysautonomia

The autonomic nervous system (ANS) regulates involuntary functions such as heartbeat, pulse rate, blood pressure, breathing, digestion and the urinary system.

Dysautonomia is a disorder that occurs when the ANS doesn't work properly, causing such symptoms as those listed below. (Note the similarity to MVPS symptoms.)

- Migraine headaches
- Spacey or dizzy feeling

- Vertigo

- Insomnia

- Hyperventilation

- Skipped or irregular heartbeats

- Raised blood pressure

- Panic attacks

- Chest pain

- Shaking or startled feeling

- Cold hands and feet

- Numbness and tingling

- Bowel and bladder problems

- Irritable bowel syndrome (IBS)

- Exercise intolerance

- Excessive sweating or not being able to sweat

- Fatigue

- Vision problems (blurred vision, vision loss, tunnel vision)

- Chronic fatigue syndrome (CFS)

- Syncope (fainting)

- Postural orthostatic tachycardia syndrome (POTS)

- Fibromyalgia

The Fight-or-Flight Response

When a person faces danger or feels fear, the body releases adrenaline to provoke the "fight-or-flight" reaction. This helps protect us and aids in survival. In the absence of any life-threatening event, the release of adrenaline often triggers my MVPS symptoms.

I have been told my anxiety triggers the adrenaline, but what if it's the reverse? What if the adrenaline is the precipitating agent that causes my anxiety and triggers the fight-or-flight response? This feels accurate. Often nothing I am doing or feeling would cause a surge in the hormone. Symptoms hit me out of the blue like a bolt of lightning. There has to be another cause for my adrenaline release.

The ANS controls our sense of well-being and can quickly change our mood from calm to panicked. If this is the case, then I am a victim of my own chemistry or, more specifically, the dysfunction of my ANS.

Two Sides of the ANS Response

The release of adrenaline from the sympathetic nervous system to help the body survive an attack has been described as being like revving a car motor or hitting the gas.

However, the ANS also includes opposing sets of nerves called the parasympathetic nervous system (PNS). Comparable to applying a car's brakes, the "rest and digest" PNS can, among other things, slow heart rate—something I can certainly appreciate.

(See: Phillip Low, MD, "Overview of the Autonomic Nervous System," *Merck Manual, Consumer Version*.)

Finding a way to calm the ANS rather than focusing on my heart and MVP seemed to be a better avenue for helpful answers, a topic I will discuss in greater detail later in this book. For now, I will say that I have never been diagnosed with dysautonomia even though I have all the symptoms. Most doctors I have seen have never acknowledged that I had MVPS much less MVPS with dysautonomia.

In his June 15, 2013, article, "Mitral Valve Prolapse – Part 6 – Getting to the Bottom of It," (MyHeart.net), Dr. Mustafa Ahmed explains that the overdiagnosis of MVP in the early days led to the consequence of adding multiple symptoms and findings to that diagnosis. Ahmed, the director of Structural Heart Disease at The University of Alabama in Birmingham, goes on to say, "Later many realized they in fact had a condition known as dysautonomia."

His opinion appears to be supported by H. Boudoulas and C.F. Wooley's findings in their February 29, 1988, research report, "Mitral Valve Prolapse Syndrome. Evidence of Hyperadrenergic State." (*National Library of Medicine*)

The report states, "The term 'MVP syndrome' (MVPS) is used to refer to symptoms due to neuroendocrine or autonomic dysfunction that occurs in patients with MVP and that cannot be explained on the basis of valvular abnormality alone."

Additionally, the researchers found that patients with MVPS showed increased levels of epinephrine (adrenaline) in urine and exhibited hyper-reactions to adrenergic stimulation such as fear.

The MVPS Diagnosis

I can understand the need to cling to the MVPS diagnosis. I feel that need, too. Nothing else seems to be generally accepted as the cause of my symptoms even if the condition is neither accepted nor well understood.

Having a diagnosis still gives me a jumping-off point to discuss my problems and look for answers. Also, I'm not sure that letting go of the MVPS diagnosis to investigate dysautonomia would be helpful as there may be a profound problem with that alternate diagnosis.

The Dysautonomia Diagnosis

In researching ANS dysfunction, I understood why no conventional doctor has treated me for dysautonomia. The current conventional thinking runs like this:

- Dysautonomia cannot be cured.

- Secondary dysautonomia will resolve when the cause is treated.

- MVPS is not considered to be one of those causes.

Doctors do not generally believe that primary dysautonomia exists except when inherited or due to a degenerative disease— which MVPS is not. That leaves me with my original diagnosis and no option for dysautonomia-specific treatment.

I have only come close to having my autonomic nervous system evaluated once. I made an appointment with a new conventional cardiologist. He was concerned with my volatile blood pressure and other adrenal complaints.

A kidney tumor, commonly a cause of dysautonomia, would have explained my symptoms.

When that test proved negative, however, the doctor completely ignored the dysfunction that alarmed him originally. I was on my own again.

In retrospect, I may have dodged a bullet. Being an outlier on the dysautonomia spectrum and not accepted by conventional medicine has protected me. Had I been diagnosed, I could have been offered potentially dangerous prescriptions used for patients who do meet the standard for treatment.

One of the drugs I researched carried a "Black Box Warning," the strictest required by the FDA when reasonable evidence exists to associate the medication with a serious hazard. All the drugs used for dysautonomia, however, come with consequential side effects.

Some of the medications used include:

- Antianxiety drugs

- Antidepressants

- Beta blockers

- Drugs that affect motor impulses

- Anti-inflammatories

- Steroids

With no cure for ANS dysfunction, these drugs could be used in combination for a lifetime to cover multiple symptoms to manage the disorder. To me, that approach seems to be similar to the drug protocol used for MVPS patients. That method exposes the patient to long-term side effects from each drug as well as potential interactions.

People with chronic, progressive, generalized dysautonomia, a condition that is recognized by conventional medicine, are considered to have a poor long-term prognosis. Death can occur from complications.

I understand that my symptoms are not as severe as people who are diagnosed by conventional medicine with dysautonomia, but why would medicine overlook other people with a milder form of ANSdysfunction? Why is it all or nothing? Many disorders are assessed on a spectrum from mild to severe.

Given the absence of a cure and the potential for serious drug risks, I feel that I am better off not being diagnosed with even a mild form of dysautonomia.

Using the MVPS/Dysautonomia Diagnosis

Even though I feel sure my symptoms result from a dysfunction of the ANS, I use the name MVPS/Dysautonomia for its familiarity.

When looking for answers, however, I am not committed to that diagnosis. While serving as a definition and ultimately validation for my problem, the term has not produced a recovery treatment. Today, I focus on the ANS to open doors to better answers.

Lifestyle changes like yoga, exercise, and the elimination of stimulants such as coffee are helpful in calming the ANS. They do not, however, treat the underlying cause of the disorder. My action plan goes deeper than useful lifestyle changes.

When a mold exposure triggered all my MVPS symptoms and caused frightening new ones, conventional medicine offered no help. Instead, I discovered a nonmedical program that taught me to take my body from a state of panic and survival to one of repair and healing. The method gave me back my life. I felt like Dorothy in the *Wizard of Oz*. When I clicked my heels, I discovered the answer had been inside me all along. (More on this in Chapter 16, Breakthrough Treatments That Changed My Life.)

The MVPS Diagnosis
Characteristic-5
Neuroplasticity and the Autonomic Nervous System

Traditionally seen as static and unchanging, it is now known that the brain adapts to new information and circumstances even after a person reaches maturity. "Brain plasticity," sometimes referred to as rewiring the brain with new neural pathways and connections, occurs when we learn new skills like using a new software package, or learning how to ski or new dance steps.

Neuroplasticity can also be used to reestablish lost abilities. New pathways can be created to bypass old or damaged ones, for instance relearning how to use an arm or a hand in the aftermath of a stroke.

(See: Dr. Pascale Michelon, "Brain Plasticity: How Learning Changes Your Brain," *Sharp Brains*, 26 February 2008.)

How Brain Wiring Can Affect MVPS/Dysautonomia Symptoms

The brain continuously learns new things and changes to adapt to new experiences. Habitual experiences reinforce performance like an athlete's ongoing training to improve his or her abilities.

Like driving a car, any repetitive action becomes ingrained until it can be accomplished without conscious thought. I can drive home every day from work, often arriving with no memory of the familiar route I used. With an understanding of that autopilot function, I asked myself if my fear reaction to chest pains had become ingrained in my brain in a similar way?

(See: Jessica Hamzelou, "Your Autopilot Mode is Real - Now We Know How the Brain Does It," *New Scientist*, 23 October 2017.)

This Is How the Theory Works

The experience of something new or scary like chest pain is sent to a portion of the brain called the amygdala. This "lizard brain" interprets the information without higher thinking. Only survival instincts are at work. The amygdala quickly sends a distress signal to the hypothalamus, which sends impulses through the autonomic nerves to the adrenal glands. Consequently, adrenaline, the chemical signaling danger, pumps through the bloodstream.

The next time the situation occurs; the brain automatically signals danger and even more rapidly initiates the same process as a means of protection. When that sequence happens in response to my chest pain, it can immediately put me into a full-blown panic.

Am I reacting to the chest pain, or has it been such a common occurrence that my brain is doing it for me? Could I break the cycle by teaching my brain a new reaction? After some work, I discovered the answer to be a definitive "yes."

(For more information on the amygdala, see: "The Amygdala," *The Science of Psychotherapy*, 21 May 2014, and James Sullivan; "Know Your Brain: The Amygdala — Unlocking the Reptilian Brain," *Brain World Magazine*, 19 April 2019.)

https://brainworldmagazine.com/know-your-brain-the-amygdala-unlocking-the-reptilian-brain/

New and dynamic programs based on neuroplasticity have taught me effective methods to rewire or train my brain. I can now stop scary reactions to inaccurate past information. (I will discuss this topic at length in Chapter 16.)

Chapter 5
Drugs: The Good, the Bad and
The Downright Deadly

The Sad Story of Two Friends

Each time a doctor prescribes a drug for me, I face the critical decision of whether to take the medication or not. A tiny pill can either improve my health and life or take both away. My frightening experiences with drug side effects, however, pale in comparison to what drugs did to two of my friends. Both died the same year.

Two different, newly released prescription drugs were involved. Each carried serious side effects. Safer drugs could have been used for their health issues, and such medications were, in fact, previously used by each of my friends without incident.

My First Friend

When a doctor prescribed a drug to my friend over the phone, he failed to consider her other medical conditions or medications. Had he done so, he would have flagged the new prescriptions as contraindicated.

When the drug failed to relieve her joint pain, he doubled the dose—again over the phone.

That was the fatal blow. Within days, the drug shut down her kidneys, causing heart failure. She died.

There were many safer treatments available for her condition, but a careless doctor with a lack of relevant knowledge killed her. A few months later, I again watched another friend die from a prescription drug.

My Second Friend

This time the culprit was a cholesterol-lowering statin. The medication, which causes devastating muscle destruction, attacked his heart, kidneys and other vital organs. Within days, his body shut down.

The drug was later taken off the market. My friend's family joined others across the United States to sue the pharmaceutical company. The drug that killed him, however, is not the only statin to be linked to a muscle-weakening effect. At the time of this writing, those drugs continue to be prescribed.

(See: "What Is Statin-Induced Myopathy or Muscle Pain?" *Healthline*, 11 July 2017.)

I try to protect myself from risks like those faced by my friends. I research drugs before agreeing to take them and, thankfully, know where to look for that information.

The PDR and Drug Inserts--It's an Open Book

Finding drug information is not difficult. Pharmaceutical companies include relevant facts in the insert packaging and list the known risks in the *Physicians' Desk Reference* (PDR).

The PDR, an annual publication, lists all drugs licensed by the U.S. Food and Drug Administration (FDA). The book provides more comprehensive information than that which is provided in the Patient Package Insert (PPI). The PPI only tells a patient how to use a drug safely. I prefer to read the inserts for professionals. I want more detailed information about the drug itself as well as its risks and side effects.

I will usually open a medical dictionary website to help me when needed as the vocabulary can be technical. I also use the website www.rxlist.com to look up specific drugs. The site, which was active at the time of this publication, provides both patient and professional information. I sometimes find it helpful to refer to both.

Additionally, I receive a newsletter from www.Drugs.com that includes drug updates, FDA alerts, drug warnings and recalls. At the time of this publication, visitors to the site could sign up for the newsletter at: https://www.drugs.com/account/register/.

What Are the Odds? What Are the Risks?

I am not against drugs. I take medications when needed, but not without prior research to determine if the prescription represents the safest and best option for my problem.

Some people do not consider the available drug information important. They think the listed side effects will not happen to them. If they're lucky, they will escape any potential harm. Sometimes odds are in the patient's favor. For example, research shows that the use of certain SSRIs, prescribed for depression, increases the risk of a stroke by one in 10,000.

(See: Press Release, "Antidepressants Linked to Increased Risk of Stroke, But Risk is Low," *American Academy of Neurology*, 17 October 2012.)

Some people may be willing to bet that they have a better chance of being one of the 9,999 people who do not suffer a stroke than to be that one lone person who does. I don't use the odds to decide whether I will take or reject a drug. I weigh the risks. For me, the risk of stroke does not warrant the use of the medication.

Unless my life is on the line and there are no safer treatments that can help, I would probably decline to take that drug.

If I become the one person to have a stroke from that drug, the risk has far outweighed the odds. What if all along there were other effective, available treatments that do not carry the stroke risk? Wouldn't that be a more viable choice?

Over the years when I have researched a prescribed drug in the PDR, I have often found that there are safer drugs available to accomplish the same goal. Armed with that information, I discussed alternatives with the prescribing doctor. On one occasion, the doctor froze for a moment in thought when I suggested a safer drug with fewer side effects. Finally, he realized that my suggestion would work as well and changed the prescription without argument.

The Problem with Drug Interactions

A drug interaction occurs when one medication affects or interferes with the function of another. According to a report in *Medline Plus*, the more drugs a person takes the higher the risk of drug interactions. ("Take Multiple Medicines Safely," *Medline Plus*.)

While most interactions are usually not life-threatening, some can lead to serious, even fatal consequences. (Leigh Ann Anderson, PharmD, "Top 9 Ways to Prevent a Deadly Drug Interaction," *Drugs.com*, 4 January 2020.)

To prevent a drug interaction, I either check with my pharmacist before taking a new drug, or I use the "Drug Interaction Checker" at drugs.com.

The Problem with Long-Term Drug Use

The chronic nature of MVPS often makes drug use a long-term proposition. The potential for side effects increases over time even if no problems are seen with initial use. According to a report by MedShadow, new research shows that taking baby aspirin for as little as three months can double the risk of macular degeneration ten years after taking aspirin.

Worse, patients may not be informed that long-term effects aren't known for many common drugs." Susanne B. Robotti, "What are Long-Term Effects of Medicine?" *Healthy Skeptic*

Heartburn drugs provide another good example of this long-term use. On many occasions I have been offered such medications for acid reflux. I am not comfortable with the potential future side effects as reported in *Science Daily*, "Popular Heartburn Drugs Linked to Higher Early Death Risk," 5 July 2017.

The article includes the following: "Popular heartburn drugs called proton pump inhibitors (PPIs), which many people take for years, have been linked to a variety of health problems during extended use. These side effects include serious kidney damage, bone fractures and dementia. A study from Washington University School of Medicine in St. Louis showed that longtime use of these drugs is also associated with an increased risk of death."

Drug Ingredients Can Change Over the Years

Some people can end up with an allergic reaction to a drug after years of taking it. This is not unusual, as discussed by Jenna Birch in the *HuffPost* article, "Surprise! Your Medication Can Have New Side Effects Years After You Start It" The article quotes Dr. Susan Besser who asserts that drug companies often change inactive ingredients like food dyes or add ingredients such as gluten.

If a person is allergic to any of these newly added substances, they may experience side effects where none were seen previously.

The One Drug I Will Take Long Term

Long-term drug use can, however, be good or even lifesaving. My father suffered from kidney damage and died of a stroke at age thirty-three from uncontrollable high blood pressure.

The first effective medications that could have saved him were not available until almost ten years after his death.

From an early age, I decided I would take blood pressure medication if I ever needed it. Another member of my family began taking a blood pressure drug in her twenties and has continued to do so for almost sixty years without issue.

As I've gotten older, my blood pressure has become an issue because of my MVPS. Most of the time my blood pressure is normal to exceptionally low, ranging between 100/ 65 to 120/80.

With an adrenaline surge, the reading can spike as high as 180/80 in a matter of seconds. I can't take medication daily, or my blood pressure will be too low. During a spike, a pill would need at least two hours to reach full effect in my system. I take my blood pressure often and use medication when indicated, but my goal is to find more effective ways to calm my ANS and control the adrenaline causing the spikes.

Some of the more helpful articles I have found that explain natural ways to lower my blood pressure include:

"8 Pill-Free Ways to Lower Your Blood Pressure," *Harvard Health Letter: Harvard Health Publishing, Harvard Medical School*, 3 May 2019.

"The 17 Best Foods for High Blood Pressure," *Healthline*, 7 September 2020.

Even though I monitor my blood pressure several times a day to help reduce my need for blood pressure medication, I still need to take a drug when the numbers go up. But, as always, there are risks.

It Happened to Me

During the initial attempt to determine the best blood pressure medicine for me, my doctor recommended a beta blocker over the calcium channel blocker I had been using.

Both drugs are used for cardiac conditions, including high blood pressure. The physician explained that calcium channel blockers dilate the arteries, which makes it easier for the heart to pump blood. But the beta blocker would block the effects of adrenaline, causing the heart to beat more slowly and with less force, which would lower my blood pressure. Controlling my adrenaline problem seemed to make sense, and I thought that the medication could potentially help my other MVPS symptoms.

I researched the drug and found health warnings I did not like but were common with this class of drugs and even with the calcium blocker I was taking. After much consideration, I decided to try the medication. I started with a very low dose and only took a third of the pill the first time.

I always take a very small amount with a new drug in case I have a negative reaction to it. Boy, was I lucky I didn't take a full dose that first time. Within thirty minutes, my whole body was vibrating and shaking. It was as if my adrenaline went into high gear and kept flowing. I thought I might be experiencing a mild seizure.

These symptoms continued for months. I tried everything to stop them. I took magnesium, B vitamins and received weekly nutritional IVs that contained a combination of several vitamins, including even more of the vitamin B family to support my nervous system.

Nothing helped.

[For more information on B vitamins. see: Carlos Alberto Calderón-Ospina and Mauricio Orlando Nava-Mesa, "B Vitamins in the Nervous System: Current Knowledge of the Biochemical Modes of

Action and Synergies of Thiamine, Pyridoxine, and Cobalamin," *CNS Neuroscience & Therapeutics*, (26:1) January 2020.]

Meanwhile, I was dropping things, slightly staggering, and losing my balance. I quivered and twitched when I tried to sleep. My teeth chattered all the time, but it wasn't from the cold.

I tried Valium, which had been prescribed to me for chronic bladder pain and found some relief. The medication quieted my body enough that I could function, and sometimes helped me sleep without twitching or jerking movements awakening me. It was a nightmare.

As months went by, I worried that the uncontrollable body movements would be permanent. I was also angry. I'd never had a good feeling about beta blockers in general. Why had I taken the prescription? The calcium blocker had been working well enough for my blood pressure, and magnesium stopped many of my other adrenaline symptoms.

Though I'd researched the beta blocker, I accepted the doctor's recommendation without listening to that little voice inside me that said, "Don't take it!"

No one, not the multitude of doctors and pharmacists I contacted, could tell me why I was experiencing the horrible side effects or what I could do to reverse them. Even the information on the drug side effects did not specifically list my symptoms, and when I contacted the drug company, they had nothing helpful to add.

A year later, the shaking, quivering and vibrating feelings slowly abated. I still don't know why the side effects subsided. But I was lucky, and I know it. I got my life back.

Occasionally, when I am unwell or physically compromised in some way, I feel that familiar shakiness, in a much milder form. Fortunately the feeling passes, but it serves to remind me that I must always be vigilant when it comes to taking drugs.

Treating Symptoms Is Not a Cure

In truth, most drugs don't really cure anything. Generally, pills address symptom relief or support body function during healing; they don't target the cause of illness. Drugs tend to be used to manage conditions such as high blood pressure. Even drugs to relieve anxiety only cover the symptoms. When a person stops the drugs, the anxiety or high blood pressure will usually return.

The exception to this assertion would be antibiotics, which kill infection-causing bacteria. Chronic infections, however, may have an underlying cause that the antibiotic does not treat. (Joseph Pizzorno, ND, "Can We Say 'Cure?,'" *Integrative Medicine: A Clinician's Journal,* 15 October 2016.)

When drugs are used to cover symptoms, the incentive to fix the underlying problem diminishes as the person feels better. For instance, reducing an individual's cholesterol numbers with drugs may not actually make that person healthier or prevent future damage. (Robert DuBroff and Michel de Lorgeril, "Cholesterol Confusion and Statin Controversy," *World Journal of Cardiology*, 26 July 2015.)

The same source notes that reducing cholesterol with drugs does not prevent heart disease but notes that the Mediterranean diet has been shown to prolong life and protect against diabetes, cancer, and coronary disease. This would seem to support my conclusion that drugs only cover a problem when there are other interventions such as a special diet that can fix it.

MVPS Drugs

Commonly used drugs for MVPS seem to fall into two basic categories: psychiatric drugs and cardiac drugs. Psychiatric drugs include antidepressants to control the emotional side of the symptoms, as well as antianxiety drugs to address the reaction to the adrenaline surges. If a person also takes cardiac drugs like beta blockers or calcium blockers, the list of drugs grows. My research shows that some of these drugs are potent, affecting or altering multiple systems in the body. In addition, taking several different drugs at once to treat various symptoms can increase the potential for drug interactions and side effects.

Another problem noted by Ronald Hoffman in *Natural Therapies for Mitral Valve Prolapse: A Good Health Guide. Keats Good Health Guides* and substantiated by my experience is that MVPS patients tend to be more sensitive to drugs in general. That sensitivity also underlies my hesitancy to take medication unless I am sure I absolutely need the drug and that it will be helpful.

I have read blogs and other postings online from people with MVPS who say they have been put on more than one drug for months but were still suffering from symptoms. After researching the most common drugs used for MVPS symptoms, I began to wonder whether the symptoms these MVPS patients noted on the blogs were because of their MVPS or because of side effects of the drugs. Or both.

A Drug Side Effect or an MVPS Symptom: Which Is Which?

Over the years, both psychiatric and cardiac drugs have been offered to me. The following list includes some of the side effects of these types of drugs. Many are eerily similar to my MVPS symptoms.

Beta Blockers

- Chest pain

- Irregular heartbeat (arrhythmia)
- Postural tachycardia syndrome (POTS)

Calcium Blockers

- Dizziness

- Fast heartbeat (palpitations)

- Fatigue

- Flushing

- Headache

- Nausea

__Antidepressants__

- Dizziness

- Agitation

- Anxiety

- Irritability

- Fatigue and drowsiness

- Insomnia

- Blurred vision

- Nausea

- Indigestion and stomach aches

- Headaches

Antianxiety Drugs

- Drowsiness

- Dizziness

- Sleep problems (insomnia)

- Memory problems

- Poor balance or coordination

- Trouble concentrating

- Irritability

- Headache

- Upset stomach

- Muscle weakness

Some of these drugs can have serious side effects on the heart. If I were to take those medications, symptoms I usually attribute to MVPS could instead be a side effect of the medications. While an MVPS symptom may be benign and not life-threatening, that same symptom as a drug side effect could be a serious warning. Given the number of MVPS symptoms, I can see how a doctor could easily dismiss an adverse drug reaction.

Drug reactions are the third-leading cause of hospital deaths in the United States. "Clinicians often misdiagnose problems caused by medications, especially when patients take multidrug combinations." (Dr. Marlene Beggelman, "Why Do We Doctors So Often Fail To See Symptoms Are Drug Side Effects?," *WBUR Boston*, 30 December 2016.)

When patients described symptoms that were known drug side effects, almost half the prescribing doctors insisted there was no connection to the medication. The impression left with patients was that the side effect was all in their head. [Beatrice A Golomb, John J. McGraw, Marcella A. Evans, and Joel E. Dimsdale, "Physician Response to Patient Reports of Adverse Drug Effects: Implications for Patient-Targeted Adverse Effect Surveillance," *Drug Safety*, 2007:30 (8).]

What Do Doctors Know About the Drugs They Prescribe?

I used to assume that doctors knew the side effects of the drugs they prescribe and would recommend only the safest and most effective medications. That is not always the case. When I began to research prescriptions rather than automatically having them filled, I discovered that in many cases I knew more about each drug than the prescribing physician.

Studies have found that many doctors don't know drug side effects at all. They have been left poorly informed by pharmaceutical representatives who concentrated on promoting drug benefits over potential risks. (Jonathan Weiss, "Doctors Don't Know The Side Effects Of The Drugs They Prescribe; Pharma Reps To Blame," *Medical Daily*, 29 May 2013.)

Who Is to Blame? Really?

I disagree with the assumption the author makes in the above-cited article. Even if a drug company representative touts the benefits of a medication they sell, doctors should know full well that there are always some drug side effects.

In my opinion, doctors have a responsibility to their patients to investigate those side effects.

All a physician has to do is take the initiative to open up the PDR and read the provided description of the medication. That due diligence would require no more than a minute or two.

For more information, see: Julia Belluz, "Why Prescription Drug Ads Always Have That Absurd List of Side Effects at the End," *Vox*, 29 September 2015.

Drugs That Get to Market Too Quickly

Even though FDA approved drug studies are considered the "gold standard" for assuring safety and efficacy, some medications are rushed to market without full testing through a process called "fast tracking."

Over a period of five years, approximately 57% of fast-tracked drugs received a "Black Box Warning," the most serious notification required by the FDA to alert consumers and healthcare providers of significant adverse effects or life-threatening risks.

(Krishnan Vengadaraga Chary, "Expedited Drug Review Process: Fast, But Flawed," *Journal of Pharmacology & Pharmacotherapeutics*," April-June 2016.)

(For more information on fast tracking and black box warnings, see: "Black Box Warnings," *Drugwatch.com*.)

Even more concerning, one-third of new drugs have safety problems even after gaining FDA approval. (Sydney Lupkin, "One-Third Of New Drugs Had Safety Problems After FDA Approval," *Shots: Health News from NPR*, 9 May 2017.")

In his article, Lupkin quotes Dr. Caleb Alexander, co-director of the Johns Hopkins Center for Drug Safety and Effectiveness: "All too often, patients and clinicians mistakenly view FDA approval as [an] indication that a product is fully safe and effective. Nothing could be further from the truth. We learn tremendous amounts about a product only once it's on the market and only after use among a broad population."

I am left to conclude that the FDA fast-track process propels drugs to market that are not well tested, putting real-world consumers in the uncomfortable role of lab rats.

As an example, let's look at the story of the drug Lotronex.

Lotronex

In February 2000, the FDA approved Lotronex to treat women with irritable bowel syndrome where diarrhea presents as the predominant symptom. This drug was offered to me, but I declined to take it.

Within months of the release of Lotronex, the drug was pulled from the market because of a significant number of deaths among women who took the medication. There were also many reported cases of ischemic colitis, a potentially life-threatening inflammation of the large intestine.

It's Back!

At the time of this writing, Lotronex has returned to the market and carries a black box warning, a caution not present when I was offered a prescription. This is one of the reasons I will generally reject new drugs in favor of older, more well-established medications that are better understood. With an older drug, I can at least find material documenting problems experienced by a large number of people over time. Aside from a faulty study protocol, other problems can affect the accuracy of drug studies.

Drug Studies: Conflict of Interest and Fraud

Potential conflicts of interest and falsified research data altered to influence the FDA approval process are also concerns with drugs new to the market.

Writing for *Science Magazine* in July 2018, Charles Piller and Jia You found potential conflicts of interest among people serving on FDA advisory panels, the groups that review drugs passing through the approval process. (See: "Hidden Conflicts? Pharma Payments to FDA Advisers After Drug Approvals Spark Ethical Concerns.")

According to Piller and You's findings, some members received significant payments from drug manufacturers or their competitors.

For more information, see: Bob Yirka, "Report Details Possible Conflict of Interest Issues for FDA Advisors," *Medical Xpress*, 6 July 2018.

Unsupervised Drugs

There may well be untold numbers of drug side effects maiming and killing the patient population because doctors are not tracking patient reactions, nor are they required to report them. These drugs appear to be used in an unstructured, non-systematic manner. Problems are usually only noted and the drug recalled after great harm has occurred.

Donald W. Light, writing for Harvard's Edmond J. Safra Center for Ethics, asserted in June 2014, "Few people know that new prescription drugs have a 1 in 5 chance of causing serious reactions after they have been approved.

 That is why expert physicians recommend not taking new drugs for at least five years unless patients have first tried better-established options..."

(See: Donald W. Light, "New Prescription Drugs: A Major Health Risk With Few Offsetting Advantages," *Edmond J. Safra Center for Ethics*, 27 June 2014.)

Patients can take the initiative to report adverse side effects on their own via the FDA's MedWatch Online Voluntary Reporting Form.

New drugs being developed today are potent and have a greater effect on the body—for both good and bad. In my opinion, these drugs are rushed to market before they are fully understood.

At least what is known about each drug is listed in the PDR. That information can help me if I need to make a decision about benefits versus risks, but that small comfort does not keep the area of new drugs from feeling like the Wild West. The following is a quick list I use when considering taking a drug:

- Research all drugs before taking them.
- Consult information on all FDA-approved drugs at www.PDR.net or www.Drugs.com or ask a pharmacist for the specific drug insert.
- Since new drugs carry more unknown risks, I always opt for older, better-established drugs.
- Avoid drugs that carry a black box warning.
- Avoid drugs with side effects similar to my MVPS symptoms.
- Weigh a drug's potential benefits against the risks and odds of suffering side effects.
- Never take drugs long term unless the problem for which they were prescribed is life-threatening.
- Remember the old adage, "Buyer beware."

Chapter 6
Choosing a Doctor: A Critical Decision

Once I filled out a survey for an MVPS support group. One of the questions asked was, "Is your doctor understanding?" I find the inclusion of that inquiry revealing. Apparently, I'm not the only one who has seen doctors who are less than understanding. It saddens me to know that being treated badly is so pervasive for people with MVPS. Even sadder still would be the revelation that the people who answered "no" were still working with an uncaring physician. Poor treatment from a doctor has always been a red flag for me, and an indicator of some of the worst care I have ever received.

To my way of thinking, choosing a doctor is the most important job I have as a patient. After working in the medical system for most of my career, I know firsthand that the choice I make can literally be the difference between life and death.

Lessons on the Dangers of Doctors

I found some sobering statistics in the HBO heart-wrenching documentary "Bleed Out." (Stephen Burrows and Judith Burrows, "Bleed Out," HBO, 2018.)

The film tells the story of how a botched surgery and recovery procedures destroyed a woman's active and independent life and left her crippled, brain-damaged and financially destitute. The documentary begins with the following terrifying list:

- 1 of 4 patients in the U.S. is harmed by medical error.
- Doctors operate on the wrong person or wrong body part 40 times a week.
- The number of patients who die from medical mistakes every year is the equivalent of three jumbo jets crashing every day.
- Medical error is third leading cause of deaths in the U.S.

Such information reinforces my belief that I must use the medical system cautiously. But most importantly, the documentary is a chilling reminder that I need to choose a doctor very, *very* carefully.

I know all too well how a doctor can determine the quality of care I receive. I have seen a multitude of doctors over my lifetime and have experienced both the best and worst of care and everything in between.

That's why I evaluate my care from my first visit and continue to reassess the doctor as time goes on. From my experience and in my opinion, I have assigned the doctors I have worked with or have seen as a patient into the following categories.

Good Doctors

Many years ago, a friend was looking for answers to her child's chronic health problem. One day she picked up a newspaper and found an article about a doctor referred to as a "medical detective" because he was able to find answers other physicians could not. His approach was to look for and fix underlying causes, and he would take the necessary time to investigate the problem.

My friend took her child to this medical detective, and over several months of treatment, he helped restore the child to health. I was intrigued. I decided to go to him myself. I was surprised to see a thick, multi-page history form of detailed questions that I had never been asked by any other physician.

After a lengthy consultation, I learned a lot about my health and the factors affecting it. The doctor helped me stay well and feel better. He was my physician for many years until he took a position in another city. The good care I received from him helped define the way I want to be treated medically. Once I realized the benefits of this kind of interaction, I could no longer settle for less. In general, I consider my "Good Doctors" to be:

- Thorough
- Open to listening to me when I bring in new information
- Willing to admit when they don't have an answer
- Willing to conduct research and confer with, or refer me to, another physician.

Limited Doctors

I cannot count how many doctors have told me their treatment was the only one that would help me. Then, on my own, I would discover the existence of other available treatments that were more effective and less risky.

These physicians are, in my estimation, "Limited Doctors." As I interpret their actions, they are either not open to alternate treatment options or feel that treatments of which they are unaware simply don't exist.

This conclusion on my part does not refer to medical specialists like gastroenterologists or neurologists. By their very nature, specialists limit their focus to their particular area of expertise. Although such physicians do not usually have answers for my chronic MVPS symptoms, they very well may still be excellent doctors in their field. I am not only an MVPS patient but also people who may have other medical issues down the road. In the future, I may need a specialist. For these reasons, I do not group these physicians with other doctors whom I see as "limited."

Conventional Doctors

I may not agree with doctors who practice conventional medicine for my day-to-day care, but I don't consider them to be bad doctors either. Several are my doctors of record, and I see them when needed. They will be there for me if I suffer an acute or critical medical problem. These are the professionals who can save my life in an emergency. They do not offer, nor do I ask them, to treat my chronic MVPS problems. Most of them have said that they have read about MVPS and are glad that I have doctors who are helping me with the problem.

I don't want anyone to think that I consider doctors who practice conventional medicine as bad. I absolutely do not. In my experience, the definition of a bad doctor, as this chapter explains, can be found in every field and every approach, including alternative medicine.

Doctors Who Blame Patients

Some doctors blame patients for their own mistakes and shortcomings. This is a well-known behavior that has been described in many books and articles.

Albert J. Miller, MD, FACC, in "Don't Blame the Patient!" [Texas Heart Institute Journal, 2011:38(6) 620] noted: "...we too often blame the patients for not getting well as they are supposed to do in response to our drugs, surgery, or various ministrations. In doing so, we close the intellectual door to seeking proper answers and diagnoses."

http://europepmc.org/article/PMC/3233310

I remember reading a book many years ago by a doctor who explained this behavior. He said that a surgeon who lost his patient after cutting a major artery told the family that the patient bled too much, and the surgical team was unable to stop it, which caused his death.

The author explained that this statement was a way of blaming the patient for excessive bleeding and not the surgeon for cutting the artery. If a doctor leans toward blaming a patient for not getting better, that physician would not be a good choice for a person like me with chronic unresolved issues.

Mean Doctors

Mean doctors are easy to spot and don't take much effort to evaluate. One doctor, on my first visit, discounted my specialized lab reports. They came from a lab that he didn't use or seem to understand. He literally threw the report back at me, calling the findings inadequate and worthless.

Another physician told me sternly that I needed to do what he recommended and stop making more out of my problems than they warranted. Then there was the doctor I knew socially who had a reputation for being a top diagnostician. Everyone recommended that I see him professionally. This was before I knew I had MVPS. I had hoped he could help me figure out why I was not feeling well. During my appointment, he yelled at me, saying there was absolutely nothing wrong with me. I'm sure patients waiting in the other rooms could hear him. I never saw him again professionally and ignored him whenever I saw him socially.

One doctor told me that I put too much pressure on him and that I made him go the extra mile. Really? He seemed to be saying he did not want to take the time, nor was he willing to look very far to help me. My good doctors will open books or go to the computer to research something and show me what they find. They go the extra mile without being asked. They do it as part of providing excellent basic care.

One of the most astonishing encounters I ever had was with a doctor who lamented that many of his patients complained too much. Well, duh! I didn't realize patients go to see a doctor for an uplifting social visit. I guess I was irritating him by talking about my health problems so I could get better and he could make a living. That was our last appointment.

When I am faced with a doctor who, in my opinion, behaves badly, I don't fight or argue. I leave and don't return. I'm not there to win a battle. My purpose is to find a good doctor and get the best care available to me.

Doctors Who Turn Vicious

A well-regarded cardiologist on staff at my hospital was kind and helpful when I had an abnormal stress test. I decided I liked him and would see him again. We had our ups and downs, but it was a relationship that basically worked for me.

I called him when I was having a nonstop flurry of arrhythmias that occurred day and night. I knew I needed another Holter monitor to find out if these arrhythmias were serious, as opposed to the results of the previous

Holter monitor test performed several years earlier. A Holter monitor is worn at home and continuously records the heart rate and rhythm for twenty-four to forty-eight hours to capture and identify dangerous arrhythmias if they occur.

I called his office and was told they could not get me in to see him for several weeks. I asked the nurse if she could get an order for a Holter monitor during my wait, and I would then have the results at my appointment. The nurse said she would set it up and would let me know. After several days when I hadn't heard anything, I tried calling again but received no return call. After almost two weeks with no response, I called my family doctor who ordered the test immediately.

To find out if there was anything specific my cardiologist would want to test, my GP's nurse called her counterpart at the cardiologist's office. The GP nurse told me later that the nurse at the cardiologist's office reacted peevishly, and defensively said, "I was working on it."

Within days, I was done with the Holter monitor. My GP got the report and did not see anything serious but recommended that I get back with my cardiologist with the results. I did. *Big mistake.* It appeared to me that my cardiologist cared more about his nurse's feelings than my situation. At my appointment, I felt his behavior toward me was abusive.

He walked into the exam room without looking at me or saying hello. He sat down, flipped through the pages of my Holter monitor report and, without looking up, blurted out, "This could be very serious. Something serious is probably causing these arrhythmias." He didn't even try to soften the blow.

I would expect that any decent doctor, even if he did not care about me personally, would deliver bad news with some kindness. It felt as if he was trying to frighten me. If so, he succeeded.

Even though my GP did not see anything alarming in the reports, I was concerned that a cardiologist might detect something the general practitioner missed. Once he delivered the scary news, he decided to take my blood pressure, which was usually a consistent 120/80 even in the doctor's office. That day, it shot up to 175/85.

The cardiologist flippantly told me, "Well, there's your cause. You could end up with a stroke or heart attack with numbers like this." I told him I never had numbers that high and asked if it could be because I was feeling very anxious about his diagnosis. He said that would not be the cause.

That was when I knew he was lying because I also knew that anxiety absolutely can make the top number spike temporarily. In no way did I think that my always low and normal blood pressure would cause dangerous arrhythmias.

I had read the Holter monitor report from my GP, and it did not show any serious arrhythmias. Even knowing that he was wrong, the cardiologist had still undermined my confidence. Once back home, I took my blood pressure. It was normal. A week later, during a visit with my GP, it was still normal. I never saw that cardiologist again and did not acknowledge him when our paths crossed.

My blood pressure remained normal for more than twenty years, and the benign arrhythmias were treated with magnesium and hypnosis, which was incredibly effective. But in my opinion, that cardiologist certainly knew how to turn into what I call a "Vicious Doctor" who not only wasn't helping but appeared to be deliberately trying to make me feel worse.

The First Time a Doctor Turned Mean

That wasn't the first time a doctor turned nasty. The first time it happened, I was in the hospital, and I wasn't able to walk away. It was during the birth of my second child. I had decided to do natural childbirth without any anaesthesia, which many mothers were doing at the time because it was considered safer for the baby.

I chose a new doctor because he promised he would help me through the birth using this natural method. Doctor support is critical to the success of this type of delivery. But the day I went into labor, he changed his mind and his attitude.

During an office visit before I went to the hospital, he said he would hook me up to an epidural, a procedure that injects a local anesthetic into the space around the spinal cord to block labor pains. Since a patient with an epidural can usually move the lower part of the body, allowing her to push during delivery, the doctor decided this method qualified as "natural" childbirth.

I declined and reminded him that I did not want any anesthesia if at all possible. He brushed me off, saying, "Well, good luck to you." I was shocked, scared and knew he was not going to help me, but it was too late to find another doctor.

My painful labor lasted all night with one contraction running into another almost nonstop, giving me no periods of relief. To make matters worse, my labor was not progressing.

The physician taking the night shift for my doctor's office was genuinely nice. It was late afternoon, and I was relieved thinking that he would be delivering my baby sometime that night.

At 7 a.m. when I was still in labor, the nice doctor came in to say goodbye. He told me that my doctor would be taking over the hospital shift. I was exhausted and in pain and scared to death.

A few minutes later, my doctor came in whistling. He seemed irreverent to me and said, "You can lie there in pain all day long, or you can get this show on the road."

With no other offer of help from him, I agreed to the epidural. He also ordered Pitocin, a natural hormone that strengthens the labor contractions to help push the baby out.

I had to sit up and lean over the side of the bed so that he could administer the epidural. The nurse held me in place while the doctor inserted a catheter into my spine to allow more doses of anesthesia if needed. He walked out while I was still leaned over, not even asking me if the epidural had taken effect.

Almost immediately, I felt severe pain in one section of my stomach. The rest of my body from the waist down was dead, something I did not expect with an epidural.

The nurse said I should not be feeling any pain and decided that I needed another dose. She called my doctor to get approval.

I was told he was drinking coffee in the doctors' lounge. Instead of coming back to check on me, he told the nurse to administer more spinal anesthesia. If he had done his job and checked before ordering more, he would have found that the Pitocin he ordered was causing the baby to come faster.

When the second unnecessary dose did not help me, the nurse told me there was nothing else that could be done for my pain. I had to endure it. My husband, who had been with me all night, suggested that the nurse check me and see the status of the baby. She begrudgingly did and was surprised, after pulling back the sheet, to find the baby's head was emerging. They rushed me to the delivery room. Although husbands were not allowed in the delivery room at that time, they let him in to help them lift me off the bed onto the delivery table.

My baby was born seconds later. Fortunately, I had an experienced delivery nurse who knew how to carefully remove the cord that was wrapped around my son's neck to bring him into this world safely.

I was then separated from my husband and baby and sent to the recovery room where there was no phone and no visitors allowed. I was all alone and could not move my body from the waist down. Later, I learned the doctor had botched administering the epidural. He'd punctured the dural that protects the spinal cord, causing temporary paralysis. Because of the unnecessary second dose, he'd approved without checking me, I remained paralyzed for more than eight hours.

When my sloppy, dangerous doctor came into the recovery room only a couple of hours later and asked me how I was feeling, I reported that I still could not move my legs. He shook his finger at me in front of everyone there and loudly proclaimed as he walked out, "If you had done what I told you to do in the first place, this would not have happened."

That's right. He blamed me for his mistake. I was to be kept in the recovery room until I could move my legs.

I watched other mothers come and go all day. As soon as I could wiggle my toes eight hours later, a kind nurse decided it was good enough and sent me to my room where I had access to a phone.

I immediately called a friend who was a nurse and asked her to contact another doctor I knew to see if he would take my case. I wanted to change physicians immediately.

The other doctor felt he could not accept me as a new patient while I was in the hospital under another doctor's care. I was stuck with what I considered to be a mean and inept physician.

As the paralysis wore off overnight, a pounding headache began. I learned later that it was called a "spinal headache," a result of the loss of spinal fluid from the fact that he had punctured the dural.

Rather than admit his mistake, the doctor did not tell me that I needed to lie flat for twenty-four to forty-eight hours to let the hole he punctured in my spine close. Untreated spinal headaches can cause life-threatening complications, including bleeding in the skull, infections and seizures.

Instead he overdosed me with a heavy pain medication that caused more problems but did nothing for the headache. When I was discharged, my head still hurt. I called a new doctor as soon as I got home, and while on the phone, he told me that I was experiencing a spinal headache and gave me directions on how to recover.

I laid flat for more than twenty-four hours, and the headache was gone. But it took weeks before my legs, left weak from the overdose of the anesthetic, finally felt stable again and for my right leg to stop buckling under me.

The fact that my baby and I recovered from the doctor's awful treatment still feels like pure luck. To this day I still believe that man's indifference and carelessness could have caused so much more damage or permanent injury. The whole ordeal certainly left me shaken, sad and angry—but it did even more than that.

The Experience Left Me Forever Changed

What happened during the delivery of my second baby was 100% the result of choosing the wrong doctor. The birth of my second child was the incident that changed my view of doctors, hospital regulations and my trust in the medical system.

I wanted to speak out and inform the public of what I had learned as a young mother at the mercy of the medical system. That experience eventually led to a career as an investigative medical reporter.

I submitted the story of my traumatic birthing experience to *D Magazine* in Dallas, Texas. The editor accepted the article in an upcoming issue.

Writing an in-depth account of my delivery helped me not only to better understand the medical system but also to heal from a harrowing experience that should have been positive.

The Power of Patients

My article, "The Baby Factory," published in *D Magazine* prompted one hospital to change its maternity department policies to support a patient-based experience rather than one designed for the convenience of the doctors. Other hospitals, in an effort to stay competitive, followed that example, demonstrating that public exposure and patient pressure can make a difference. That was when I realized that, as a journalist, my reports could expose problems within the medical system, inform and empower patients to protect themselves, and serve as an impetus for change. We can't fix what we can't see. In large part, my ignorance of the lenient hospital policies governing the doctors on staff allowed, and perhaps helped to cause, what my child and I had faced—the unnecessary risk and pain.

Provoking Change

In my experience as a medical reporter, I have continued to see patients' demands generate sufficient energy to turn the tide. A large number of unhappy consumers protesting by voice, vote, or purchasing choice can propel a situation to its tipping point.

What I require as a patient may improve my care, but when other patients also demand an improved experience, the result can force sweeping changes that benefit everyone—including future patients. My *D Magazine* article introduced me to the power of public exposure and patient pressure to quality of care. See: "The Baby Factory," *D Magazine*, September 1978.

Lesson Learned

That experience taught me to choose my doctors with great care. Today I will not hesitate to leave a doctor who shows any signs of unkindness or lack of understanding. This behavior indicates to me a forewarning of possible worse behavior to come.

There are too many good doctors I can choose instead of jeopardizing my care by staying with an insensitive doctor in the hope that the doctor will change.

Past Changes Patients Have Made

When I was younger, patients were not allowed to see or copy their medical records. That policy kept patients in the dark and allowed doctors to maintain control. In one of my reports about medical record access, I used the example of money.

Would customers deposit money in a bank and give away all decision-making power? The financial institution would decide how the funds would be invested if they could be spent, and grant or deny the account holder access to account statements. The answer? Of course not. Denying patients access to medical records felt equally crazy to me, yet people accepted the policy without question, ceding access to critical information about their health.

I left the care of any doctor who would not give me copies of my medical records. At the time, they had a right to deny access to me, but it was always followed by the assertion that I would not understand the material the records contained, a common excuse used back then.

To circumvent that denial, I would change to a doctor who would give me copies of the records, and then have the uncooperative physician forward all my files to the new doctor. In the end, I got the records anyway, and I had no problem understanding their contents or accessing any help I needed to interpret the information. The entire process to me seemed like nothing more than a power play.

Who Owns My Medical Records Anyway?

At the time, I had to play those games as doctors actually owned their patient records. If a physician died, the records passed into the possession of the doctor's heirs. I had a friend whose therapist died. Her husband inherited all the records from her practice, including my friend's records and the personal information they contained.

The husband refused my friend's request to relinquish the records, assuring her that the material would be safely stored in his garage. Who knows what happened to those files when he died?

As ridiculous as this may seem today, the practice was completely acceptable in the late 1980s—a time period that hardly qualified as the Dark Ages. This begs the question, is there anything occurring in medicine today that is equally ridiculous? Questioning old practices considered common seems like a good idea to me, especially at times when the medical system is not working well for me.

Patient Referrals

Receiving a physician recommendation from a friend doesn't always work out either. When I asked a good friend for a referral to a gastroenterologist to get an opinion on a lingering pain following my gallbladder surgery, she recommended a doctor she said she loved. I found the man to be condescending, testy and quick to offer an unnecessary procedure.

He reviewed my history, but instead of addressing my pain, he became more interested in my acid indigestion issues, which were under control and not bothering me at the time. The doctor wanted to biopsy my upper GI tract to look for signs of gluten intolerance. I asked him what he would prescribe if he found the problem. His reply? A gluten-free diet.

Why would a physician subject a patient to an invasive procedure if the proposed treatment could also be used as a risk-free diagnostic tool? If I went on the diet and felt better, problem solved.

When I brought up the reason for my visit again—the unresolved pain—the doctor became annoyed, an indication to me that there would be worse behavior to come. To redirect his interest away from my upper GI issues, I told him I had not eaten gluten in more than fifteen years, something he never asked.

I gave him one last chance to address my postsurgical stomach pain. He barely examined me and then blew me off, saying the discomfort would probably get better on its own. The visit was a waste of my time. I'm sure he felt much the same way as he did not get to perform his recommended procedure. A physician my friend considered to be the most wonderful doctor ever was, for me, not even a good one. I saw warnings of future bad behavior in his response to me. While a recommendation can be helpful, in the final analysis, my best decision came from a single factor—how that doctor treated me.

Insurance Companies vs. Fee-for-Service

Many of the doctors I see are "fee-for-service." They do not take insurance; therefore, I pay for the services I receive. Otherwise, the insurance company would dictate my care, deciding which treatments and medications qualify for reimbursement under the terms of my policy.

Sometimes I need to pay out of pocket to get the best doctor for my health issues. For example, when I suffered numerous daily arrhythmias, my "fee-for-service" doctor ordered a magnesium challenge test which revealed that I was deficient in that mineral.

Bringing my magnesium levels back to normal stopped almost all the arrhythmias. That protocol was not reimbursable by my insurance company, but a less accurate blood test would be, therefore, most doctors would have ordered the blood work. Had a doctor prescribed a beta blocker for my arrhythmias, the insurance company would have paid—but not for intravenous magnesium or injections of the mineral. *(See: Chapter 7: Magnesium: The Remarkable Mineral and How I Use It.)*

Also, doctors on most insurance plans are not sufficiently reimbursed for each visit to spend time with me. For financial purposes, they need to see as many patients as possible. A quick visit with a doctor will not help me. I don't come with problems that are easy to diagnose or treat.

For the times I need the more standard or usual treatments, I see doctors who are covered by my medical insurance, like a dermatologist to treat a rash. In the end, whether the insurance company pays or does not pay will not determine what doctor I see or what treatment I accept.

Although I don't have unlimited funds, I am fortunate to have enough income—and the willingness to prioritize healthcare over other expenses—to pay when needed. Paying out of pocket means I receive the treatment my physician thinks best rather than those the insurance company will cover.

Doctor Overview

MVPS patients come with a perplexing and unusual mixture of symptoms that can be resistant to treatments. I can certainly understand that every doctor I see will not necessarily have answers for me, but I need to be careful when searching for a new doctor that I avoid and hopefully never inadvertently hire any of the limited, mean or vicious ones.

Part II
My Action Plan

Chapter 7
Magnesium:
The Remarkable Mineral and How I Use It

Note

This chapter contains information gained from medical professionals, personal research, and personal experience. I am not an expert on magnesium. I have, however, benefited from the knowledge of experts. Readers can, if they choose, use the citations in this chapter to conduct their own research. People with any health problem, especially people with kidney issues should check with their doctor before taking magnesium or any other supplement.

Magnesium

The human body requires magnesium for more than 350 biochemical processes. Magnesium helps to regulate blood pressure, maintain strong bones, and ensure a steady heart rhythm.

The mineral helps to relax nerves, muscles, bronchial tubes, and blood vessels. This effect explains how magnesium can help to relieve:

- migraines, which are vascular spasms in the head
- arrhythmias, which are vascular spasms in the heart
- IBS, which are spasms in the colon.

Magnesium has been referred to as "Nature's Valium" because the mineral's overall calming effect is a natural therapy for anxiety.

What happens when a person has a magnesium deficiency? The answer was, for me, a familiar list of symptoms that made the mineral an essential part of my action plan.

Magnesium Deficiency or MVPS Symptoms?

The magnesium deficiency symptoms listed below read like a list of MVPS symptoms. I don't know if magnesium deficiency causes my MVPS symptoms, but I can attest that magnesium, in the right dose, using the right protocol, has helped to reduce those symptoms significantly. I feel much better in general when I take magnesium regularly and worse when I do not.

In Natural Therapies for Mitral Valve Prolapse: A Good Health Guide. Keats Good Health Guides., Dr. Ronald L. Hoffman notes the same association: "It's been estimated that as much as 40 percent of the population of the industrialized nations suffer from magnesium deficiency while at the same time, 85 percent of people with mitral valve prolapse appear to have some magnesium deficiency.*"

The following is a list of the more common, less serious symptoms of magnesium deficiency.

Many are the same as those listed for MVPS. This familiar list of symptoms raises the question, "Are all my symptoms caused by MVPS or caused by a magnesium deficiency?" An asterisk indicates that it is one of my MVPS symptoms.

Symptoms of Magnesium Deficiency:

- Migraines*
- Irregular heartbeat*
- Numbness or tingling in your extremities*
- Anxiety*
- Depression
- Irritability
- Vertigo*
- Sleep problems*
- Muscle weakness, twitches and cramps*
- Fatigue*

- High blood pressure*
- Asthma
- Seizures
- Poor appetite
- Nausea*
- Sleepiness*
- IBS*

Magnesium and Mitral Valve Prolapse

Although magnesium deficiency symptoms mirror the symptoms of the MVP "syndrome," MVP itself is an identifiable heart condition. My earliest tests showed a mitral valve that billowed when it closed. While still a benign condition, I believe that anything that strengthens the heart is essential to my health. According to many reports, magnesium is a therapy that can do that.

James J. DiNicolantonio, Jing Liu and James H. O'Keefe, writing for *BMJ Journals*, cited magnesium as both a preventative and treatment for cardiovascular disease that "plays an important role in cardiovascular health."

The conclusion of the article asserts that magnesium deficiency can lead to serious morbidity and mortality and has been implicated in multiple cardiovascular diseases such as hypertension and cardiac arrhythmia. (DiNicolantonio, Liu and O'Keefe, "Magnesium for the Prevention and Treatment of Cardiovascular Disease," *BMJ Journals: OpenHeart*, 2018.)

Magnesium and Heart Attacks

A British study of more than 2,300 patients also indicated that magnesium may reduce deaths from a heart attack by as much as 25%. The author noted that in the United States, where magnesium is not standard medical care for cardiac patients, approximately half of the one million Americans who suffer a heart attack each year die as a result.

(S.M. Horner, "Efficacy of Intravenous Magnesium in Acute Myocardial Infarction in Reducing Arrhythmias and Mortality. Meta-analysis of Magnesium in Acute Myocardial Infarction," *Circulation*, 1 September 1992 86:3.)

Magnesium and the Sister Syndromes

Magnesium is also implicated in other medical problems, including the MVPS sister syndromes, fibromyalgia and chronic fatigue syndrome/myalgic encephalomyelitis (See: Chapter 4: Five Conflicting Characteristics of the MVPS Diagnosis and How Knowing Them Has Helped My Treatment)

Fibromyalgia

Research published in *Rheumatology International*, an independent journal on rheumatic diseases, points to an association between magnesium levels and fibromyalgia symptoms.

The study by Omer Faruk Sendur, Engin Tastaban, Yasemin Turan, and Cevval Ulman found significantly decreased serum levels of magnesium in fibromyalgia patients. The researchers concluded that serum magnesium may play an important role in the pathophysiology of fibromyalgia.

[See: Sendur, Tastaban, Turan, and Ulman, "The Relationship Between Serum Trace Element Levels and Clinical Parameters in Patients with Fibromyalgia," *Rheumatology International*, 28 September 2008: (11).]

A second article in *Nutrients*, a peer-reviewed journal of human nutrition, pointed to the ability of magnesium to alleviate the symptoms of fibromyalgia, dysmenorrhea, headaches, and acute migraine attacks. [Hyun-Jung Shin, Hyo-Seok Na, and Sang-Hwan Do, "Magnesium and Pain," *Nutrients*, 23 July 2020: 12(80).]

Chronic Fatigue Syndrome/Myalgic Encephalomyelitis

A study in the United Kingdom showed magnesium improved symptoms of chronic fatigue syndrome/myalgic encephalomyelitis (CFS/ME). "Patients treated with intramuscular magnesium sulfate for six weeks had higher self-reported energy levels, better emotional state and less pain on the Nottingham Health Profile when compared to a placebo."

(See: I.M. Cox; M.J. Campbell, PhD; and D. Dowson, MB, "Red Blood Cell Magnesium and Chronic Fatigue Syndrome," *The Lancet*, 30 March 1991.)

The Right Dose Matters

In my opinion, the underuse of magnesium reflects a lack of knowledge on the part of many doctors about how to prescribe the mineral. I have seen this reflected in conversations I've had with many conventional doctors, including cardiologists, about the use of magnesium.

If they approve of me using the mineral—and many of them do not—they recommend a low amount roughly in line with the recommended daily dose of 420 mg/day for men and 320 for women in my age range. I have never experienced any significant improvement in my MVPS symptoms at that low dose. To me, the recommended dose amounts to being instructed to take half an aspirin a day for a migraine.

When I experience MVPS symptoms like arrhythmias and migraines, the only effective treatment to stop either has been an IV of 2,000 milligrams of magnesium or an injection of 1,000 milligrams.

(Please note that those cited amounts do not constitute a recommendation on my part but merely reflect the amounts that have been administered to me in the past under the care of a physician.)

When my symptoms subside, I have been able to maintain my magnesium levels by taking between 500 to 1000 milligrams a day orally—again as per my doctor's recommendation.

(For more information, see: David Larson, M.D., "Magnesium, the Magic Mineral," *LifeWellness Institute*, 8 June 2018.)

Loose bowels is the only adverse reaction I have ever experienced from the oral use of a magnesium supplement. I would liken the effect to that of taking a mild laxative. In fact, the mineral is used in Milk of Magnesia, well known as a gentle laxative. Simply cutting back on the dose of the mineral resolved the issue.

Using the RDA daily recommendation of magnesium instead of a therapeutic dose to treat symptoms may be why many doctors do not consider the mineral to be an effective treatment for arrhythmias. Instead, they will recommend a calcium channel blocker, something I have been offered many times for my MVPS symptoms. According to a published research study by Mark Houston MD, MS, "Magnesium is a natural calcium channel blocker."

(See: Mark Houston, MD, MS, "The Role of Magnesium in Hypertension and Cardiovascular Disease," *The Journal of Clinical Hypertension*, 26 September 2001.)

This assertion makes sense to me. Calcium and magnesium compete for the same receptor sites within cells that receive signals and initiate responses. The more magnesium that is onboard could serve to block the effects of calcium on the cells. ("Receptor: Definition and Function," *Study.com*.)

Calcium channel blockers are drugs that work by slowing the movement of calcium into the cells of the heart and blood vessel walls. The heart can then pump blood more easily through the widened vessels. ("High Blood Pressure and Calcium Channel Blockers," *WebMD.com*, 24 September 2019.)

Both calcium and magnesium are needed for balance, however. Magnesium helps the heart muscle cells relax by countering the calcium which stimulates contractions. These minerals compete with each other to ensure heart cells contract and relax properly. ("What Does Magnesium Do for Your Body?," Healthline.)

Given these facts, why would I want to block calcium with a drug when adding more magnesium will achieve the same effect naturally and help balance out the calcium? In addition, magnesium carries multiple benefits and none of the side effects of a calcium channel blocker.

In my case, the more important consideration is that magnesium has proven to be the only treatment to improve some of my worst MVPS symptoms.

Oral vs. Injectable Delivery

Receiving magnesium intravenously or as an injection allows the mineral to be more directly absorbed into the body. I can feel the effect within minutes, which is not the case when I take an oral supplement.

Oral medications are broken down by stomach acids before passing through the liver and into the bloodstream. The effectiveness of the drug can be altered by physiological factors, such as gastrointestinal pH, gastric emptying, small intestinal transit time, bile salt, absorption mechanism and other factors.

With all my stomach problems, I have no idea how much of the magnesium is actually absorbed when I take a supplement by mouth.

See: Nai-Ning Song, Shao-Yu Zhang, and Chang-Xiao Liu, "Overview of Factors Affecting Oral Drug Absorption," *ResearchGate.net*, September 2004; and "How Does The Body Metabolize Medication?," *Orlando Clinical Research Center,* 26 September 2016.

There are some precautions when using magnesium—for instance, those with kidney problems should not use the mineral. There are also some other potential side effects. See: "Magnesium," *WebMD.com*. However,

hypermagnesemia or high magnesium levels is rare because the kidneys work to get rid of excess magnesium. This problem is most often seen in people with poor kidney function.

Finally, be aware that all commercially injectable magnesium contains aluminum, which has been associated with neurological problems. My doctor uses a specifically compounded form of the mineral that does not contain aluminum.

Getting Magnesium from the Diet?

Some professionals have suggested that I eat more magnesium-rich foods. That strategy can be good for the diet in general, but in my case, it has not elevated my depleted magnesium levels or helped to reduce my symptoms.

I don't see how it could be humanly possible to eat enough magnesium-rich food in a day to make an appreciable difference in my levels. One doctor suggested I consume foods with added magnesium.

It should go without saying that I have no desire to attempt to get my magnesium from eating processed, synthetic foods infused with a potentially inferior form of the mineral. In addition, I only eat unprocessed, organic foods, and I only use high-grade magnesium manufactured by quality labs that have been recommended by my doctor or by a nutritionist at a reputable health food store.

How Do I Know When I Am Low in Magnesium?

There are tests to measure magnesium levels. However, the typical blood test run by my conventional doctor did not show a deficiency. The test only tabulates the amount of magnesium in the blood at a specific moment in time, not whether the mineral is reaching the bones, cells, and tissues. Generally, approximately 1% of total body magnesium is present in the blood. ("Magnesium," *LabTestsOnline.com*, 6 December 2019.)

According to the National Institute of Health, evaluating magnesium levels with blood serum presents problems. Levels of the mineral found within cells and bone present little correlation to total body levels.

Serum magnesium can also tell a false story because when magnesium in heart cells declines, the body tries to compensate, thus elevating the serum levels—meaning, high levels of magnesium in the blood may actually signal an overall deficiency. (Ronald Grisanti D.C., D.A.B.C.O., D.A.C.B.N., M.S, "Magnesium: The Fact That Can Kill You," *Functional Medicine University*.)

In my opinion and based on my experience, the magnesium challenge or magnesium load test, which uses urine, returns greater accuracy. Sources suggest that many experts consider this method to be the preferable means of measurement.

(See: "Magnesium," *National Institutes of Health: Office of Dietary Supplements*, and DiNicolantonio, Liu and O'Keefe, "Magnesium for the Prevention and Treatment of Cardiovascular Disease," *BMJ Journals: OpenHeart*, 2018.)

I Did the Magnesium Urine Challenge Test

Over twenty-four hours, I collected urine prior to receiving two injections of magnesium calibrated to my body weight. After the magnesium injection, I collected urine over another twenty-four-hour period. The body will excrete any magnesium it does not need. The goal of this test is to see how much magnesium my body retained, which would indicate how much my body needed. Analyzing levels before and after the injections allowed for those calculations to be made. Retention of more than 20% would signal a magnesium deficiency. My body absorbed almost all of the injected mineral. The two test injections I received made me feel better immediately yet a blood test the week before returned normal levels.

Replenish and Then Maintain

When my magnesium level drops, oral doses do not help rebuild it. I need to reestablish my levels with IVs or injections. Once established, it can be maintained through diet and supplements.

Research agrees with this protocol. [Brent N. Reed; Su Zhang, J. S. Marron; Deborah Montague, "Comparison of Intravenous and Oral Magnesium Replacement in Hospitalized Patients with Cardiovascular Disease," *American Journal of Health-System Pharmacy*, 2012: (69) 14.]

Bottom line, for me, this treatment provides significant improvement in my symptoms almost immediately. The benefits can last for months or longer if I do not deplete my magnesium levels again.

What Causes Magnesium Depletion?

Many factors can deplete magnesium levels. Some can be controlled, but not all. I do find, however, that there are ways to at least lessen many of their effects.

Factors that deplete magnesium include:

- Stress
- Chronic disease
- Pain
- Gastrointestinal problems
- Hyperthyroidism
- Alcohol
- Diuretics
- Some medications
- Age (absorption decreases with age)
- GI problems (interferes with the ability to absorb magnesium)
- Adrenaline and cortisol (cause the release of magnesium from cells that are lost through the urine)
- Diet (the typical American diet lacks magnesium because of farming practices)
- Carbonated beverages
- High levels of calcium supplements
- Diabetes
- Kidney dysfunction

Specific conditions in women that deplete magnesium include:

- Pregnancy
- Nursing
- Estrogen levels
  (which are affected by PMS and menopause)

Foods that Help Increase Magnesium and Foods That Don't

These are the foods I use in my diet to help maintain my magnesium levels.

Helpful Foods

- Nuts and seeds
- Whole grains
- Fish and seafood
- Beans
- Spinach
- Avocados
- Bananas
- *Foods I Avoid*
- Gluten
- Refined sugar
- Soft drinks
- Alcohol
- Nonorganic foods
- Salt

Magnesium Alert

I wear a medical alert bracelet that lists my allergies along with a list of drugs that I can safely take in case of an emergency. I have added to the instructions that I be given magnesium IVs should I have a cardiac event. I can only hope that I get a good doctor who is up to speed on the benefits of magnesium if I am not able to speak for myself.

For more information on magnesium, see:

- Emily Laurence, "How You Can Use Magnesium to Help With Migraines, IBS, and Anxiety," *Well+Good,* 15 November 2017.
- "Magnesium Sulfate for Asthma Treatment," *Medical News Today*, 20 November 2018.

- "Magnesium Fact Sheet," *National Institutes of Health, Office of Dietary Supplements*, 25 September 2020.

- Atli Arnarson, "7 Signs and Symptoms of Magnesium Deficiency," *Healthline*, 15 December 2017.

- Dr. Lindsey Berkson, "Magnesium is Nature's Valium," *drlindseyberkson.com*.

- Mark Hyman, M.D., "5 Simple Steps to Cure IBS Without Drugs," *drhyman.com*.

- Afshin Samaie, Nabiollah Asghari, Jafar Ard, et al, "Blood Magnesium Levels in Migraineurs Within and Between the Headache Attacks: A Case Control Study," *The Pan African Medical Journal*, 2012: 11(46)

Chapter 8
Be Still My Heart:
How I Calm and Stop Arrhythmias

Arrhythmias can take my breath away, leave me light-headed and make me feel like someone did a karate chop behind my knees. No matter how those episodes affect me, or how scared I may be, every doctor I've consulted describes them as "benign"—except one.

Benign or Life-Threatening

During a routine stress test, the nurse started to complete the procedure, saying enough information had been collected. I said I didn't feel completely stressed and asked to push further. She agreed.

Out of the blue, I felt a familiar thud in my chest. It didn't affect me, so I kept running. The nurse, however, noticed something on the EKG, stopped the treadmill, laid me down on the table and started the echocardiogram.

A staff person ran out of the room. Moments later one of the doctors in the clinic opened the door and asked if I had any signs of a cardiac problem. Huh? The nurse answered, "No."

After I got dressed, the doctor told me my arrhythmia registered 11 on a scale of 1 to 10. The EKG showed that I had a V-tach, a ventricular tachycardia, which is life-threatening and can stop the heart in an instant. People with V-tach require an implanted defibrillator that sends out a forceful shock to stop the dangerously fast rhythms or, if needed, restart the heart.

My test happened on a Friday afternoon. The cardiologist scheduled a cardiac catheterization for the first thing Monday morning. During the procedure, a thin tube is inserted into an artery and threaded through the blood vessel to the heart.

Doctors use the test to diagnose and treat cardiovascular conditions. The cardiologist told me to go home and rest, but if I experienced more arrhythmias over the weekend, I should check into the hospital immediately.

After an irregular EKG ten years earlier, I underwent a cardiac cath that showed no problems. This one, however, was more concerning because the doctor had identified a specific and dangerous problem.

While I waited for Monday, I researched the condition but could not find a reason for V-tach that was not serious and life-threatening. I called my regular doctor. He had always been able to help me with my MVPS symptoms.

 On several occasions he saved me from what was thought to be a potentially serious problem by finding that the actual cause was benign.

With regret, he told me he did not have a protocol for this type of arrhythmia and advised me to stay the course with my cardiologist. I think that was my lowest moment.

I've always found a way out of a scary prognosis and a way back to health by finding someone who would address the underlying issue. That option didn't seem open to me for dealing with V-tach.

Finally, I contacted my cousin who works in the medical field. She listened and thought that her friend, a medical director at a major California cardiac center, might have a better treatment. She left messages all weekend asking if I could fly out for a consultation but did not hear back from him. Monday morning came. On the drive to the hospital, I continued to hope he would call, but that didn't happen.

The cardiologist met me in pre-op and tried to prepare me for the eventuality of a serious problem. I kept asking if MVPS could be the cause.

I believed then, and believe now, that MVPS caused the irregular EKG that prompted the first cardiac cath a decade earlier.

The cardiologist responded that the cause of the V-tach wouldn't matter. I would still need a cardioverter defibrillator (ICD) to save my life from future episodes.

I knew that implanting a defibrillator would also end my life as I had known it. Once the device has been implanted, the patient can no longer drive because both the arrhythmia and the resulting ICD shock can cause fainting. My independence would end, and I would live with the lurking threat of a dangerous arrhythmia that scared me more than any MVPS symptom ever did.

When I awakened from the cardiac cath, the cardiologist told me the results were perfectly normal, but an electrophysiologist, a specialist in arrhythmias, would meet with me later that day. The doctor went on to say that the failure to find an underlying cause did not change the fact that I had a dangerous arrhythmia that required treatment.

I was to stay in the hospital overnight, and the next day the electrophysiologist would implant the defibrillator. My cousin waited with me in the hospital room where, finally, the sound of her phone ringing broke the silence. The California cardiologist finally called her back. He had been out of town all weekend. He recommended a protocol that could be done at a local clinic where I lived or said I could come to his center and go through his program. His treatment, which would address the cause of the V-tachs, would remove the need for a defibrillator. Since he had successfully treated many patients with the identical problem, I decided to do his program.

I was ready to leave the hospital that day no matter what was recommended. When the arrhythmia specialist came in, I was prepared to tell him that I was going to forego more procedures, go home, and think through my options. He beat me to the punch. I had what he called a rare, benign V-tach and was free to go home. I don't remember anything else he said except to make an appointment to see him after I recovered from the cardiac cath. He is still my doctor to this day.

The nurse arrived to help me check out. I can still see the surprise on her face as she gave me a congratulatory hug for the good news I'd received. Apparently, it was uncommon for V-tach patients to go home without an implant.

As I dressed and packed my belongings, I wondered if the whole frightening episode wasn't just another false alarm—a common occurrence in my life since I began dealing with MVPS. I have continued to have other V-tach arrhythmias on my EKGs and have been told by other cardiologists reading the reports that they follow an electrical pathway that does not lead to my heart. Therefore, they are considered harmless.

Bottom Line

The medical profession either ignores me, labels me a hypochondriac, or over diagnoses dangerous cardiac events, which after extensive testing turn out to be nothing serious. These frightening episodes are documented, entered into my file, and become the baseline for what is normal for me.

To me, however, these scary events do not feel unrelated. The doctors I see try to find a cause for each symptom as if it stands alone. Although they cannot find any causes, none of these physicians are willing to consider the only constant in my medical history as the culprit—MVPS.

My Arrhythmias

Many people, even those who do not have MVPS, experience benign arrhythmias. ("Heart Rhythm Disorders," *Upbeat.org*.) However, there are several types of arrhythmias, some serious and life-threatening.

I always check with my doctor when arrhythmias feel different or change in any way I find concerning. To date, I have not had any dangerous arrhythmias except for the single V-tach episode, which in the end was found to be benign.

Catching Arrhythmias

When my arrhythmia began, I expressed concern to my doctors. I felt a thumping in my chest as if my heart skipped beats or beat too rapidly. At times I even felt light-headed.

I received typical 30-second EKG monitoring while lying on the exam table before being told my heart was fine. One doctor grew frustrated with me, pointing out that

I had just undergone my first cardiac catheterization, reminding me the procedure found nothing abnormal.

In response, I asked how the cardiac cath could evaluate my heart rhythm if the problem was not happening at the time of the procedure. I was not given any helpful response. Several months later I found a new doctor who finally ordered a Holter monitor, which identified a variety of frequent, benign daily arrhythmias. After finally having been validated, I began the magnesium treatment that helped to calm my heart's rhythms.

How My Arrhythmias Feel

The first time I felt an arrhythmia I did not know I had MVPS. The flutter in my chest lasted no longer than a second with no other accompanying symptoms. Over time, the fluttering would not stop until I coughed or breathed out quickly and forcefully. If I didn't react quick enough, I would feel a little light-headed.

I still experience those kinds of arrhythmias but not often. Sometimes I can feel my heart pulsating through my body, especially in my throat and neck.

Other times, the sensation is one of pounding in my chest or the skipping of a beat. These events do not interfere with my life and occur only rarely now.

Most of my arrhythmias consist of premature atrial contractions (PACs) and premature ventricular contractions (PVCs), which are considered benign. Sometimes they occur in a series of every two beats called bigeminy or every three beats called trigeminy.

These can be problematic, but in my case, I experience such runs only occasionally, and they do not represent a threat to my health. Over the years, my health has improved. The last time I wore a Holter monitor for thirty days, the device detected no runs and very few arrhythmias.

What Can Cause My Arrhythmias and How I Treat Them

Several factors and instances can trigger my arrhythmias, but I have developed strategies for preventing them.

Low Magnesium

I try to keep my magnesium levels in a normal range, increasing the dosage when presented with a flurry of arrhythmias. This has always helped. To me, the success of the intervention indicates that low magnesium could be the most apparent cause of the irregular heart rhythm. My doctors agree.

Electrolyte Imbalances

Electrolytes are minerals, such as sodium, potassium, calcium and magnesium, that are found in the body. Low electrolytes can cause multiple symptoms including irregular heartbeat, fast heart rate, and fatigue. Once a year or at any time I feel symptomatic, my electrolyte levels are checked with a simple blood test. Other than magnesium, my electrolyte levels have been normal.

Stress

Stress, anger, and depression have all been shown to have a significant impact on cardiac arrhythmias. [Una Buckley, MD and Kalyanam Shivkumar, MD, PhD, "Stress-Induced Cardiac Arrhythmias: The Heart–Brain Interaction," *Trends in Cardiovascular Medicine*, 2016 January: 26 (1).]

Stress can also deplete magnesium, but frankly, that factor constitutes something of a chicken or egg dynamic. Stress lowers my magnesium level, or the low level causes my stress—circular conundrums I resolve by simply knowing that I need to both reduce my stress and increase my magnesium.

Adrenaline Primer

Endogenous adrenaline, also called the stress hormone, is produced within the body and is released to protect a person from danger. It's sometimes called the "fight-or-flight" hormone. Other factors, such as stress, excitement and even diet can activate the release of adrenaline, which can cause:

- rapid heart rate
- rapid breathing
- increased blood pressure
- sweating
- jittery or nervous feeling
- heightened senses

(See: "Adrenaline Rush: Everything You Should Know," *Healthline.com*.)

The release of adrenaline in my body can trigger many of my MVPS symptoms, including arrhythmias and chest pain. If I react to the symptom with fear, even more adrenaline may be released. This double dose of the hormone can increase the intensity of my symptoms and make me feel even worse. There are methods to stop that second flood of adrenaline and the higher level of anxiety, which I will address in Chapter 16.

Epinephrine (Adrenaline as a Drug)

Epinephrine, which is used in medicine for many different purposes, is an external source of adrenaline. Since adrenaline produced in my body has been a source of many of my MVPS symptoms, I do not want to add epinephrine if I can avoid it.

Common adverse reactions to epinephrine are similar to endogenous adrenaline (produced inside the body) and include:

- anxiety
- apprehensiveness
- restlessness
- tremor
- weakness
- dizziness
- sweating
- palpitations
- pallor
- nausea
- vomiting

- headache
- respiratory difficulties

No thanks.

Epinephrine in the Dentist Office

Epinephrine, as a drug, is used in dentists' offices to keep Novocain in the injection site longer by constricting the blood vessels in the deadened area. Blood vessel constriction causes my migraine headaches and the accompanying stroke-like symptoms.

Because I refuse the use of epinephrine, Novocain often wears off for me before a dental procedure has been completed, requiring additional injections. I prefer that to provoking my MVPS symptoms.

Before I understood the combined use of epinephrine and Novocain, I would feel many of the adrenaline's effects including shaking while waiting for my injection to take effect. One dentist accused me of simply being nervous about the procedure. I was not and told him so. Still, he continued to blame my emotions instead of recognizing the side effects of the epinephrine he administered to me.

When I learned I was reacting to the epinephrine, I made changes to my medical history. When filling out a history form with new doctors,

I always include epinephrine on my list of allergies. I also notified my existing doctors to add that information to my files. The drug is now flagged as an allergy on all of my medical records.

I also found a new dentist I could trust to take my symptoms seriously and who had a better grasp of the side effects of the drugs he uses and prescribes.

Not Just the Dentist Office

During a dermatologist appointment to remove a spot, I refused to agree to the use of epinephrine and Novocain in combined form to deaden the area. I assumed the procedure would have to be rescheduled, but the doctor used a different method, injecting fluid to expand the location prior to cutting. I felt no pain and avoided the side effects of epinephrine. I did not, however, have similar good luck with an ophthalmologist.

In that instance, the ophthalmologist did not check my flagged allergies before using eye drops for dilation that contained epinephrine. My blood pressure shot up almost immediately, and I began to shake.

The tech in the room didn't know how to use the automatic blood pressure monitor, so I did it for her. The numbers were high, prompting the doctor to return and stay with me until the situation began to resolve.

He checked my eyes as soon as possible and sent me on my way— and he apologized. I drove home carefully, but I was wiped out for hours with a migraine and the unsteady, spacey feeling it causes. And yes, I have a new ophthalmologist.

I didn't leave him because he failed to review my chart. Anyone can make a mistake. I left because he hired a tech who was unable to take my blood pressure—or find anyone in the office who could help her to do so. If a mistake is made in a clinic, I do at least expect the requisite level of competency to be present to address it.

The Benefits of Epinephrine

To be fair, epinephrine can treat life-threatening allergic reactions to insect bites, food allergies, and adverse drug reactions. Some people have to keep epinephrine with them at all times.

The drug can also stop bleeding in cases of traumatic injury. There may be a time when I will need epinephrine, but

in optional cases, the medication isn't good for me and can cause arrhythmias.

Hypoglycemia (Low Blood Sugar) Can Cause Arrhythmias

For me, hypoglycaemia or low blood sugar (glucose) can trigger MVPS symptoms, including arrhythmias and migraine headaches. Low blood sugar can occur when I eat too much sugar, do not eat enough protein, or do not eat often enough.

Hypoglycemia and Too Much Sugar

People who feel hypoglycemic fatigue during the day will often say they need a quick pick-me-up, which usually means eating a food high in sugar. That strategy isn't the best idea with MVPS.

When sugar enters the bloodstream, insulin enters as well, grabbing the sugar and carrying it to the cells for use. This rapid process can leave insufficient sugar in the bloodstream, resulting in low blood sugar or hypoglycemia. The body then releases adrenaline to raise blood sugar levels, which, in my case, triggers MVPS symptoms *and* adverse adrenaline symptoms. That is why I avoid sugar. Refined carbohydrates like white rice, pasta and bread rapidly break down into glucose in the body just like a sugary food, so I avoid eating those items except in combination with protein.

Hypoglycemia and Not Enough Protein

Protein helps stabilize and sustain blood glucose (sugar) levels. It also helps slow down the digestion of carbohydrates, reducing spikes in blood sugar after meals.

Eating protein at every meal and for snacks can usually keep my blood sugar levels steady all day. I eat a protein snack before bed to prevent morning hypoglycemia, which is caused by not eating for an extended period overnight. When this happens, I can wake up light-headed or with a headache. If adrenaline kicks in to elevate my blood sugar, I can also start my day with one or more of my MVPS symptoms.

Hypoglycemia and Not Eating Often Enough

Blood sugar comes from the food we eat and is used for energy. When blood sugar levels are too low, the body becomes starved for energy. To help provide the needed energy, the body releases adrenaline to raise blood sugar levels.

This can also trigger my MVPS symptoms. Hypoglycemia causes hunger and shakiness. If I am dealing with the symptoms of both, I can be left feeling hungry and shaky with a migraine headache and arrhythmias—all at once.

Eating some protein every three to four hours throughout the day has turned out to be an easy way to keep my blood sugar levels even and prevent a flare-up of my MVPS symptoms.

Chemical Sensitivities

Artificial chemicals can trigger my MVPS. Such sensitivities are listed among the symptoms for the condition, but many people without MVPS experience such negative reactions, especially to toxic substances derived from petroleum products.

In its online guide to "Unknown Chemical Exposure," the Virginia Department of Health states: "A small chemical exposure can cause tearing eyes along with burning of the eyes, nose, throat, chest and skin. It may cause headache, sweating, blurred vision, stomach aches and diarrhea."

Exposure to a toxin can also cause me to suffer an allergic reaction that releases histamine and, in turn, adrenaline. The body cannot handle large amounts of histamine, which adrenaline counters.

Histamine causes:

- hives
- itchy skin
- red eyes
- facial swelling
- runny nose
- congestion
- headaches
- or asthma attacks.

When I end up reacting to both the adrenaline and the histamine, I can feel pretty miserable after an exposure to toxic chemicals. Artificial fragrances and insecticides are the most toxic to me, causing arrhythmias and migraine headaches. Additional symptoms may include light-headedness, dizziness, spaciness, and shakiness. I try to avoid any exposure to chemicals and I do not purchase or use them.

The Allergy Treatment That Helped

Unfortunately, I cannot always avoid exposure to toxic chemicals or offending foods. For this reason, I use allergy drops prescribed by my doctor after I underwent specialized "provocation/neutralization" allergy testing.

The half-day test involved the injection of one allergen at a time under the skin to provoke a reaction. All resulting symptoms are noted. When a reaction occurs, weaker doses are progressively administered until the symptoms stop. That neutralizing dose then becomes the designated treatment. I put the specially formulated drops under my tongue twice a day and after any exposures that cause symptoms.

Diet can also affect heart rhythm. Caffeine and some herbs act as stimulants. Additionally, food allergies can affect the heart and can cause the histamine/adrenaline release cycle. As an example, I stay away from monosodium glutamate (MSG), a flavor enhancer often found in Chinese foods and some processed foods. MSG has been banned from my diet for more than thirty-five years, since I realized that it causes migraine auras and triggers other MVPS symptoms.

Eating Can Cause a Pounding Heart

The act of eating changes blood flow increases heart rate and raises blood pressure. Overeating forces the heart to work harder than normal because the digestive process requires more blood to be pumped.

Sugars and high-carbohydrate foods lower blood sugar, which can cause heart palpitations. Salt may have a similar effect on the heart's action along with spicy or rich foods that cause heartburn.

See: "What Causes Palpitations?" *Healthline.com.*

How I Treat Arrhythmias

If I cannot prevent arrhythmias by controlling my magnesium levels, diet, allergies and stress, I have strategies that work to reduce or stop the episodes. Some are common methods, while others are strategies I discovered on my own. All are sufficiently helpful that I keep a list for my reference.

A Word About the Vagus Nerve

The vagus nerve is an important part of the parasympathetic nervous system. The nerve runs from the brainstem through the neck and upper chest down to the abdomen. Unlike the sympathetic nervous

145

system that responds to adrenaline to prepare a person for a "fight-or-flight" situation, the parasympathetic nervous system helps the body relax and recover more quickly following stress. Stimulating the vagus nerve stimulates the parasympathetic nervous system, which can reduce heart rate and blood pressure and can help the body to relax. See: Jordan Fallis, "How to Stimulate Your Vagus Nerve for Better Mental Health," 21 January 2017.

See: Sigrid Breit, Aleksandra Kupferberg, and Gregor Hasler, et al, "Vagus Nerve as Modulator of the Brain–Gut Axis in Psychiatric and Inflammatory Disorders," *Frontiers in Psychiatry*, 2018 (9) 44.

Unsigned educational PDF "Vagus Nerve" from Rice University.

(Note: The second referenced source was available at the time of this publication and, to my knowledge, can only be accessed at the provided link. For readers of the paperback edition of this work, the full address is: www.caam.rice.edu/~cox/wrap/vagusnerve.pdf.)

Some issues, however, can have a negative effect on the vagus nerve, including GI distress and hiatal hernia, both of which I have. Poor posture, along with muscular imbalances, can also cause the vagus nerve to misfire, as can excess alcohol or spicy foods. The nerve is also subject to irritation from stress, fatigue and anxiety. (Jill Blakeway, MSc, LAc, "Using the Gallbladder Divergent Channel to Calm an Irritated Vagus Nerve," *Pacific College of Health and Science.*)

Compromised vagus nerve function can cause symptoms including but not limited to:

- Nausea
- Heartburn
- Vertigo
- Tachycardia (accelerated heartbeat)
- Irregular or accelerated heartbeat

- Headache
- Fainting

In cases of persistent arrhythmia, I use cold water to both drink and splash on my face. Because the vagus nerve is connected to the vocal cords, singing, humming, or even gargling can also provide helpful stimulation. ("Voice & Swallowing - Anatomy," *OHSU: Ear, Nose and Throat, ohsu.edu.*)

There are times when I feel like I need to throw the book at the problem and do everything all at once. No matter what I do; however, remaining calm to prevent additional adrenaline release until my heart calms is essential.

For more information, see: "What Is the Valsalva Maneuver?" *WebMD.com.*

Drink Water

I learned that drinking adequate amounts of water helps the heart. Dehydration thickens the blood, slowing down circulation and forcing the walls of the blood vessels to constrict as they struggle to work. To compensate, the heart beats faster, causing an increase in heart rate and palpitations. Alcohol consumption aggravates the problem by causing or worsening existing dehydration.

I am sensitive to electromagnetic fields. The issue doesn't bother me enough that I am forced to shut down anything around me that generates such a field, but I can feel the effect from time to time. For instance, I stopped wearing my smartwatch because the device caused a tingling sensation along my arm even when no notifications or calls came in. I have chosen to follow the advice offered by earlier researchers on the relationship between electromagnetic fields and heart function: "Until the effects of EMF on heart tissue are more fully explored, electronic devices generating EMFs should be approached with caution."

See: Onur Elmas, "Effects of Electromagnetic Field Exposure on the Heart: A Systematic Review," *Toxicology and Industrial Health*, 10 September 2013.

With this in mind, I will sometimes be cautious and shut down my computers, television, Wi-Fi, wireless devices and cell phone, and not use my cordless phone while going through a flurry of arrhythmias.

Additionally, I sometimes walk outside barefoot on dirt and grass to connect with the earth. This "grounding" or "earthing" is thought to help many people with healing a variety of health issues. The premise holds that today we are disconnected from the earth because our shoes and flooring prevent the planet's natural energy from reaching our bodies. Perhaps the transfer of the earth's electrons from the ground to the body explains why so many people find walking on the beach such a pleasurable experience.

Some health professionals think that "earthing" can have a positive effect on the autonomic nervous system (ANS), heart rate variability (HRV), and blood viscosity (thickness). The simple, natural process has no side effects, and I like how it makes me feel.

Gaétan Chevalier, Stephen T. Sinatra, Pawel Sokal, et al, writing in the *Journal of Environmental and Public Health*, said: "emerging scientific research has revealed a surprisingly positive and overlooked environmental factor on health: direct physical contact with the vast supply of electrons on the surface of the Earth. Modern lifestyle separates humans from such contact. The research suggests that this disconnect may be a major contributor to physiological dysfunction and unwellness. Reconnection with the Earth's electrons has been found to promote intriguing physiological changes and subjective reports of well-being."

(See: Chevalier, Sinatra, Sokal, et al, "Earthing: Health Implications of Reconnecting the Human Body to the Earth's Surface Electrons," *The Journal of Environmental and Public Health*, 2012.)

Other Actions Have Helped:

- Place a cold cloth on my face and pressure points
- Use a fan to blow air on my face
- Gently and continuously pat my diaphragm under my ribs
- Put magnesium under my tongue to get it into my system faster
- Put sublingual vitamin B complex drops under my tongue
- Lie down and elevate my legs
- Change positions; turn over to the other side
- Walk around and stretch
- Watch my posture; I sit up and open my chest instead of slumping
- Slow down breathing to about six breaths per minute especially on the exhale.
- Meditate and visualize myself calm and feeling good
- Remind myself that the arrhythmias always stop, so I should stay calm to prevent the release of more adrenaline

I have read that acupuncture, osteopathic manipulation and yoga can help. I have used all three for other issues successfully and will try them in the future if needed.

The Best Nondrug Treatment I Have Ever Used

A friend of mine recommended a psychologist on staff at the University of Texas Southwestern Medical Center, a medical teaching facility in Dallas, who used hypnosis for patients undergoing surgery. The psychologist was successfully helping people before and after procedures to feel less anxiety, recover faster and need less pain medication.

He worked with my friend's mother to visualize health while she was receiving treatment for terminal lung cancer. This psychologist's therapy was part of the protocol that put her cancer into remission.

I made an appointment with him when my arrhythmias were out of control and gave me no peace. An elderly gentleman with a comforting manner, he incorporated my description of my symptoms along with his suggestions in his therapy.

He made a tape of our session for me to use as often as needed. I saw him several times for more sessions to solidify the therapeutic effects. For years, I never felt another arrhythmia. Once, a doctor listening to my chest told me he heard skipped beats, but I did not feel them.

I felt liberated from the symptoms. When they started to creep back in, I made another appointment to stop them again. Even though he has since passed away, I learned the power of hypnosis from him and continue to benefit from its use. I have developed my own audio recording based on my current situation that employs more powerful suggestions that seem to work even better for me.

Since I know that my arrhythmias are not serious, I do not worry when I get them. Instead, I use the methods I noted above to resolve the episode. I also try to prevent such incidents by treating my allergies, stomach issues and low magnesium levels. It is this information that has helped me be able to stay calm and act more effectively when dealing with arrhythmias and all my MVPS symptoms.

Chapter 9
"Phantom Heart Attack"
Identifying, Treating, and Stopping
Noncardiac Chest Pain

Disclaimer:

I am not advocating that anyone else use my approach to decide if and when to go to the ER with chest pain. Chest pain can be serious, if not deadly, when not treated immediately. I absolutely know that to be true. That is why there are guidelines for when people should go to the ER. These guidelines include a list of symptoms that indicate the probability of a heart attack. I personally know people who waited too long and lost their lives because they made that mistake.

However, I have come up with strategies at home that have helped provide me with information about my body when I have chest pains. Over the years, I have been to the emergency room numerous times to find out that my chest pains are not caused by a heart attack or any cardiac issue.

My last checkup with my cardiologist was completely normal, and I was told that all tests showed that my heart is strong and healthy. Still, that has not stopped occasional chest pains.

Today, when I have what feels like my typical chest pain, I do not immediately run to the ER. Instead, I can use my tools and strategies to help identify and treat any of the other health issues I have been diagnosed with that can and do cause chest pain.

I also take into account my medical history which includes two normal cardiac caths, a low level of plaque as seen on my cardiac computed tomography (CT) for calcium scoring, a generally low blood pressure level, a normal echocardiogram and benign types of arrhythmias. Knowing all of this has helped me make decisions about when to seek medical attention, but in no way do I think it is foolproof. Everything I do has risks and benefits, and I don't know which wins out until I have hindsight. When I choose not to go to the ER, I know I am taking a calculated risk.

The following is only an example of what I do and why I do it whenever I have chest pain.

My decisions have absolutely nothing to do with anyone else's specific situation at any given time, nor am I recommending my system to anyone to use.

The information and descriptions provided here are an example of an action plan I made for myself as a nonmedical professional using all the data I have collected about my unique health profile. My methods were not developed for anyone else's medical situation.

Chest Pains

When working at a medical school in the News and Information Department, I did a radio series for heart month that ran on the Texas State Network. One episode included an interview with an ER doctor.

He explained that many people with chest pain have died because they did not want to come to the ER in case their symptoms were a false alarm. The physician made his position clear. "Come to the ER and let us make that determination. That's what we are here for."

Ten years later I did what he recommended when my MVPS chest pains confused my mind and body. I became a regular at the ER, racing there to get reassurance. The problem for me was that the chest pains did not feel the same each time, so I could not get a baseline. As a result, I kept going back to the ER to let the doctors evaluate each new or different kind of pain.

The chest pains seemed to reinvent themselves with each occurrence. Each time, I was found to be okay, and each time my complaints lost a little more of their credibility.

My Body Speaks to Me in Riddles

My chest pains always seem to mimic a heart attack. I asked myself, what is my body trying to tell me? Something serious or nothing at all? I realized that I was using the ER in an effort to interpret those communications. I wanted to know what my body was saying to me in case it was serious, but I could not make the determination alone. Nor could I use the American Heart Association's warning signs for women that indicated a heart attack. Why? Because I experienced all of the listed symptoms on a regular basis except for vomiting. The listed warning signs are:

- Uncomfortable pressure, squeezing, fullness or pain in the center of your chest. It lasts more than a few minutes or goes away and comes back.
- Pain or discomfort in one or both arms, the back, neck, jaw or stomach.
- Shortness of breath with or without chest discomfort.
- Other signs such as breaking out in a cold sweat, nausea or light-headedness.
- As with men, women's most common heart attack symptom is chest pain or discomfort.
- But women are somewhat more likely than men to experience some of the other common symptoms, particularly shortness of breath, nausea/vomiting and back or jaw pain.

See: "Heart Attack Symptoms in Women," Heart.org.

Rosie O'Donnell's Heart Rap

Rosie O'Donnell, an American comedian, actress and television personality, almost died because she did not realize she was having a heart attack. After her recovery, she set out to educate women on the telltale symptoms. The rap song she created may be the most helpful for me as these are not symptoms I usually experience, so they could signal something more serious should I ever have them.

Rosie lists of symptoms are:

- Hot
- Exhausted
- Pain
- Pale
- Puke

Her rap version of the symptoms helps people to remember the list. At the time of this publication, the clip from her comedy special was available on YouTube and at other sites by searching online for the phrase "Rosie heart attack rap."

A second YouTube clip, also available at the time of this publication on the user channel "Dominique V," included a portion of the comedy special explaining in greater detail what Rosie experienced during her heart attack.

Where is the MVPS List?

Although the American Heart Association's warning list of symptoms for a heart attack might be helpful for others, they are not to me. Those same symptoms have prompted me to go to the ER numerous times when nothing was wrong.

Where is my list, the one that tells people like me with MVPS when I should go to the ER?

Rosie O'Donnell's list is more helpful because she explains what she felt, which I can relate to better than a clinical list of symptoms.

Still, Rosie did not have any of those symptoms before her heart attack. They did not hound and confuse her for years as my symptoms have. She knew the sensations were not the norm for her. But the classic symptoms of a heart attack are common to me.

When I decide not to go to the ER, it is not because I am in denial but because I am confused. I ask myself, what can I do at home to responsibly assess my symptoms? I want to be able to objectively evaluate if what I am feeling are my normal, benign symptoms or something more serious that requires medical attention.

Undoubtedly doctors will say that I should not take matters into my own hands and that such a response could be dangerous. They're right. It is a risk. But what should I do when a patient like me is discounted for coming to the ER too often with a false alarm? I can either go to the ER and be given a prescription for Valium and sent home or be chided for staying home when it could have been a heart attack. To make the decision even more complicated, I am also discouraged from finding a way to assess my problem while at home on my own.

My body cries wolf over and over again, which makes me feel like I have no choice. Hundreds of times over the past twenty years I've chosen not to go to the ER with scary chest pains. To date, I've never had a heart attack. At my last annual checkup, my cardiologist found my heart to be strong and healthy.

I remember a time when doctors discouraged home blood pressure monitoring with equipment easily available today. They reasoned that patients wouldn't know what to do with the information they collected. We now understand that home monitoring not only improves the quality of care for patients but has been lifesaving. I am not inclined to stay in the dark and be barred from the information I need to take care of myself.

Since I don't have a helpful list from the American Heart Association to tell me when I, with all my confusing symptoms, need to seek medical care, I feel I need home tools that can help me come to that conclusion on my own.

How About a Team Effort?

If doctors do not like patients to carry this tremendous weight on their shoulders, then maybe they could help people like me make that determination at home.

It would be life changing if I could check my heart remotely with a physician who could evaluate the results and let me know if I should go to the ER. Home testing would eliminate doubt and danger.

This is not wishful thinking. In my research, I located such a device in development by researchers at the University of Turku, Finland. Their technology would allow the use of a smartphone's built-in motion sensors to detect a myocardial infarction or heart attack. ("New Smartphone App Detects Heart Attacks," *Diagnostic and Interventional Cardiology*, 28 October 2016.)

Still Waiting...

That 2016 article projected testing for the technology in 2017. If this device is already in use or if there are any other remote testing devices or apps available, they should be in widespread use, easy to find by patients and offered by doctors.

Heart disease is the leading cause of death in the United States, with one person dying every 37 seconds. A device like the one developed by Finnish researchers could save lives. It would certainly help me make a more accurate decision about what to do anytime I have chest pain.

I would stop worrying that I am making a mistake by either staying home or going to the ER. For now, however, I remain on my own, with no one to help me in reaching that decision.

To Go or Not to Go, That Is the Question

I don't rush to the ER as quickly as I once did. I'm not embarrassed by the prospect of the doctors finding nothing wrong, but I am concerned that repeated false alarm visits will cause me to be discounted for a future serious cardiac event.

This is not an unfounded concern. Several times I have felt the judgment of ER doctors as they reviewed my medical file and noted my frequent ER visits for the same complaint. Such conversations almost always end with the offer of antianxiety medication.

As a further complication, women are frequently discounted even in instances when they are suffering from a heart attack. Sometimes even during a cardiac event, a woman's EKG will appear to be normal. Doctors need to always take women seriously, hold them for observation, and run specific tests to help diagnose a heart attack. However, that doesn't always happen. I know that if I am discounted, my symptoms may not be accorded the weight they deserve.

(See: Jessica Firger, "Why Do Doctors Ignore Signs of Heart Attacks in Women?" *New York Post*, 26 February 2018.)

Even so, it would be foolish to sit at home paralyzed with fear waiting for a chest pain to resolve or become so severe my health and life are in jeopardy. Unfortunately, that was all I knew to do before I developed a reliable action plan.

Idly waiting and worrying only caused the release of more of the adrenaline that likely caused my symptoms in the first place. That single hormone always makes my chest pain—and everything else— worse. Discounting the release of adrenaline doesn't work either, because the hormone does have important benefits. There is always the chance that the hormone was released to signal something serious.

Adrenaline may be released as a protective response, decreasing the body's ability to feel pain. This reaction would allow a person to keep running or fighting danger even in the presence of an injury. The hormone might very well keep a person alive until they can access medical care.

(See: "What Happens to Your Body During the Fight or Flight Response?," *Cleveland Clinic: Health Essentials*, 9 December 2019.)

This is another reason why I believe I need to do something other than to sit at home and worry. If I have an action plan, I'm busy evaluating my chest pain. That helps to keep me calm. Clearheaded action, instead of passive fear, can prevent the release of more unnecessary adrenaline, which can often help improve the symptoms. I also know that if I see anything concerning, I will seek medical care.

My Chest Pain Action Plan

My chest pains from MVPS get my attention whether they come on quietly or abruptly. Since I have other medical issues that could also cause chest pain, I have a two-pronged system to try to figure out the cause for each episode.

1. I check and monitor my heart. Any problems on that front will send me straight to the ER. Since I started using this system, there has been no need to seek medical aid for a cardiac issue.
2. I treat the other potential causes of my chest pain at the same time. If the treatment works, the pain stops and the cause is revealed.

How I Monitor My Heart

In addition to watching for any common symptoms listed by the American Heart Association and Rosie O'Donnell's list, I have three main tools that tell me how my heart is functioning. These are the same tests that would be done upon arrival at the ER.

EKG Home Unit

The resource chapter at the end of the book includes a list of the EKG models I have used. This is, however, a moving target. No sooner does a unit come on the market than it will vanish entirely or carry the ambiguous "not available" tag. I saw a home EKG unit for the first time on the *Today Show* more than twenty years ago and purchased it immediately. Apparently the company sold out quickly. Later, when I tried to purchase a backup unit, none could be found.

Over the years, I have read articles in newspapers and magazines featuring doctors critical of the use of home EKG machines. These physicians could not see patients using the technology in a safe, positive way, going so far as to suggest such a practice would be dangerous. They took the position that only a doctor can accurately check heart function, harkening back to the days when patients were not allowed to see their medical records for similar reasons. If I don't understand something, I ask for help or look it up. I don't like doctors who keep me in the dark while making decisions for me.

When that first EKG machine broke, I called the wholesaler to order a replacement. The distributor told me that they were still selling in other countries but not in the United States because of new FDA red tape. That seemed to support my suspicion that the medical community's pressure to keep the device out of the hands of patients succeeded.

I learned that if an item could not be purchased in the United States, I could order it from other countries or ask friends traveling abroad to purchase it for me. In my opinion, products sold in countries like

Canada, the United Kingdom, Japan, or Israel will be of equal quality to those available in the United States. Therefore, I have no concerns about accuracy.

Today, however, technological advances have given the public applications that run on smartphones that seem capable of performing almost any task. Patients can now buy user-friendly, reasonably priced EKG models that relay a great deal of information regardless of the user's ability to read a conventional EKG tracing strip. One well-marketed unit comes with a specific limitation.

The patient buys the device. The reports are sent to a doctor for interpretation. This could be a good option for some people, but I don't want such an arrangement to be my only option.

My EKG units produce printouts that I can take to my doctor or forward to his office via email. I prefer that with my EKG unit I can know in the moment if something is wrong and go to the ER, and I can share the readout with my personal physician later.

I choose units on the market that can be purchased without a prescription and can provide the necessary information to me without an intermediary. I am the only one who needs that data immediately. Currently I have both a primary and backup EKG unit.

Understand that these home machines are for reference only. They record, but they do not diagnose, nor are they as comprehensive as the machines used in a medical setting. I do find the devices to be helpful, however, to spot-check for irregular heartbeats and to help indicate when something has changed or does not fall within my normal readings. If I have any symptoms that are concerning to me, I seek medical attention no matter what my EKG unit says.

Blood Pressure Monitor/Cuff (Sphygmomanometer)

Next, I take my blood pressure. When I have adrenaline on board, my blood pressure will spike a bit, but I do need to know if the numbers are higher than usual, a potential signal of a cardiac event. If the reading is elevated, even slightly, I work to bring the levels back to a normal range. In the event of spikes or any other concerns I might have, I will take a prescribed calcium channel blocker. My blood pressure generally runs low to normal.

I only take the medication when the reading spikes over 140/80. I also use calming techniques, some used for arrhythmias, (See Chapter 8) that will lower my BP during adrenaline-related episodes. More on this in Chapter 16.

Manual Monitor with Inflation Bulb vs. Automatic Monitor

There are two types of monitors available: automatic and manual. I have both that I will sometimes use in combination to get more accurate numbers.

Automatic Monitor

Over time, I have found that the automatic monitor can give me numbers out of my normal range or that are questionable for the given situation. When this happens, I recheck my blood pressure with the manual unit after waiting a couple of minutes.

I always have the option to contact the manufacturer for advice in adjusting an automatic unit when it's consistently inaccurate. If repairs aren't possible, I buy a new monitor.

I regularly take both monitors to any doctor's appointment to check their accuracy against the clinic's readings. If the devices are not too far off, I continue to use them at home. If, however, a reading is way off, I replace the unit with a new one.

My preference is to use an arm cuff. I dislike wrist models because they never seem to provide the same level of accuracy.

Manual Monitor with Inflation Bulb

Manual units are difficult to use, but I do prefer their accuracy. The devices require that I put my arm in the cuff, adjust the flat side of the stethoscope chest piece under the cuff, and then put on the stethoscope earpieces. I place the bulb in my right hand and hold the meter in the other hand, on the arm where I placed the cuff. The pump requires strength, but I try to remain relaxed. Good light is essential to read the meter, especially at night.

Because my upper number can spike as high as 180, I pump up the pressure to 200 and then slowly let out the air. For me, this method is not as quick or as easy as using the automatic unit, but the results are more consistent with the readings taken in my doctor's office.

Pulse Oximeter

Whenever I have gone to the ER for chest pain, following a blood pressure evaluation, my oxygen levels are checked with an inexpensive device called a pulse oximeter. I bought one of the devices, which clips onto the index finger, for home use. The display also shows pulse rate. Anything under 100 is considered normal, but I like to see my rate around 60, which is normal for me.

Oxygen levels should fall within a range of 95%-100%. Anything under 90 is considered low and is referred to as "hypoxemia." This could indicate an issue with breathing or circulation. Shortness of breath is a common symptom of hypoxemia. If my oxygen levels are above 95%, my pulse is below 100 and I am not panting for air, I consider the readings to be in line with what is normal for me. I continue to repeat all three of these tests until the episode passes.

My Treatments

Baby Aspirin

Among my first actions, I chew four baby aspirin. This is recommended at the first signs of a potential heart attack as it can slow clotting. Taking it can also help alleviate pain even in the absence of a heart attack. Although I did have a stomach bleed years ago when I took high doses of aspirin four times a day for a twisted ankle, the one-time, low-dose baby aspirin is good insurance and worth the risks. I've had no stomach issues with this protocol.

ER GI Cocktail

Because I have GERD (gastroesophageal reflux disease), my chest pains could be caused by the flow of stomach acid into the esophagus where the tissue can become inflamed and painful. If I suspect this to be the case, I mix and drink a GI cocktail.

The mixture is identical to the one given in the ER to differentiate between GERD-related chest pain and a cardiac event. Because I have prescriptions for lidocaine and the sedative Donnatal, used for stomach pain, I can make the cocktail at home. I mix the two drugs with a liquid antacid. I rarely have to resort to this remedy, but when I do, it can help stop the chest pain and help identify GERD as the possible cause.

Bentyl

When my IBS causes painful cramps, I take the antispasmodic medication Bentyl (generic name dicyclomine). The drug slows the gut's natural movements by relaxing the stomach and intestinal muscles. Additionally, Bentyl can relieve spasms in the upper stomach connected to the esophagus.

The esophagus connects the throat with the stomach and runs behind the heart. "A diaphragm spasm is a sudden, involuntary contraction that often causes a fluttering feeling in the chest. It is also common to experience a temporary tightness in the chest or difficulty breathing during the spasm." ("Diaphragm Spasms and Flutters: What to Know," *Medical News Today*, 3 January 2020.)

IBS is also caused by visceral (inner organs) hypersensitivity and often occurs in people who have no cardiac chest pain. ("Visceral Hypersensitivity and IBS," Very well Health, October 24, 2020)

I also have a hiatal hernia, a condition in which the upper part of the stomach bulges through an opening in the diaphragm. I can feel the hernia under my ribs. A hiatal hernia can cause:

- heartburn
- stomach pain
- diaphragm spasm
- chest pain radiating down the arms and back up to the neck

Radiating pain of that nature is also a symptom of a heart attack, but when it is caused by a hiatal hernia, it does not typically cause additional alarming sensations like shortness of breath, chest tightness, sweating or nausea. Bentyl usually relieves these GI spasms fairly quickly. With so many possibilities for cardiac-like symptoms that are not heart related, it is no wonder MVPS patients can be confused.

Osteopathic Manipulation, Pain Medicine and Heat

Costochondritis, an inflammation of the cartilage between the ribs and breastbone, further complicates my stomach problems. The pain caused by this condition also mimics cardiac conditions and heart attacks. ("Costochondritis," *The Mayo Clinic*, mayoclinic.org.)

I have used osteopathic manipulation to treat the problem, which helps, but the relief does not last. Home massage techniques can help release the tightness between the ribs.

Placing the heels of my hands on both sides of the rib cage, I simply press each side back and forth to get the movement within the affected area. Upper body stretches, trigger point massage, and yoga—anything that introduces mobility at the site of the restriction—have been of benefit to me. Baby aspirin helps reduce or stop the rib pain, but a heating pad or warm, moist heat from a Bed Buddy® offers immediate relief and can even lessen GERD-related chest pain.

Heat also calms my nervous system, which in general reduces the level of discomfort.

Staying Calm

These measures give me something productive to do, countering worry and helping me to understand what my symptoms may actually mean. Also, I am never alone, even when I am. I wear a medical alert button, a device that is not just a protection for older people at risk of falling. I've used one of the devices since I was in my thirties for times when I am alone. Now it's easy to buy an inexpensive device that operates with a smartphone or can call a landline. Additionally, I keep a cordless phone with me at all times. These precautions lower my anxiety level.

For me, taking precautions prevents worry. The story of thirty-one-year-old Jonathan Metz of Connecticut has stayed with me. In 2010, Metz, who lived alone, went down to his basement to adjust the heat. His arm became caught between two heating cores inside the boiler.

Metz had no phone or any other means of communication. No one heard his cries for help or looked for him. After three days, the trapped man smelled rot setting into his crushed arm.

Realizing the onset of a life-threatening infection, Metz used his tools to amputate the arm and save his life. (Russell Goldman, "Man Trapped in Furnace Amputated Own Arm to Live," *ABC News*, 11 June 2010.)

Had he worn a monitor or carried a phone, Metz might not have lost his arm. My monitor will detect if I fall. I don't even need to be conscious to get help. The response team has my history and my contacts.

Although I have never needed to rely on the device, having it makes me feel more secure. Anything that keeps me calm and prevents worry appears to keep my adrenaline levels from spiking.

Sick as a Dog and Healthy as a Horse

Living with MVPS has given me a life of contradictions. In addition to the "MVPS Phantom Heart Attack," I also experience a large number of symptoms and maladies that would make most people think that I am either neurotic or at death's door.

Even though I have:

- chronic migraines with stroke-like symptoms
- vertigo
- fibromyalgia
- joint and muscle pain
- various kinds of arrhythmias
- hypoglycemia
- IBS
- anxiety
- a bunch of other very unpleasant sensations

I am not sick. No matter how bad I feel, I am basically healthy and very grateful when I get a clean bill of health with each checkup.

As I Get Older

The older I get the greater the chance that my chest pain actually could signal an actual cardiac event. I am at that age where women face a greater risk of a heart attack. That fact is on my mind every time I have, what has been to date, benign chest pains.

I get regular EKGs at my doctor's office and watch my blood pressure. I have also had a CT angiography, a heart CT scan using X-rays of the heart and blood vessels to detect any buildup of calcium.

My vessels are clear, and I have been told that at my age, they will probably stay that way. My last echocardiogram showed my heart to be quite strong.

I am fortunate. Still, as I age, even with my action plan, I cannot completely rule out a serious cardiac event whenever I have chest pain. With the help of my tools, experiences and a general understanding of the signs of a heart attack, I now have more sources of information to help me determine the necessity of an ER visit.

Still, the conventional wisdom cautions against waiting. I have seen what can happen if a person doesn't act. Recently, a friend who spent the day with chest and stomach pains rejected his wife's suggestion to go to the ER for an evaluation. He remained in denial for more than twelve hours until late that night when those subtle symptoms roared and literally stopped him in his tracks. His wife called an ambulance, but it was too late.

I'm not in denial. Instead, I'm a person with MVPS trying to be responsible and calm in the face of confusing and recurring chest pain. However, if I become at all concerned, I won't hesitate to seek medical help.

Chapter 10
My Migraine Headache Protocol:
Aura, Pain and Stroke-Like Symptoms

At age forty-two, I was diagnosed with my first migraine headache. The frightening incident sent me to the ER with tingling down one side of my body, inside my mouth and down my throat.

After learning the sensations signaled a migraine, I realized I had experienced variations of the symptoms most of my life without realizing it. Since I didn't know how to describe what I had felt, I kept the episodes to myself. The tingling down my side, however, was new and a common warning sign of stroke.

Subsequent research indicated I have symptoms of two types of migraines: hemiplegic and brainstem aura. These have included:

- Dizziness
- Vertigo
- Nausea
- Spacey-unreal feeling
- Sensitivity to light and sound
- Tingling
- Weakness
- Visual symptoms

The visual manifestations take several forms:

- A crescent shape obstruction in one eye
- Multiple small spots scattered across the visual field
- Flashes of light

My migraines typically manifest initially with fleeting dizziness or light-headedness with one large, gray spot in my peripheral visions. Within minutes, the other symptoms begin.

The weird sensations worsened when I started taking birth control pills in my early twenties. I knew something had changed, but I tried to ignore it. One night, however, while visiting with friends, an episode overwhelmed me. For the entire night,

I functioned in a dream state where nothing felt real. I struggled to be social and pretend I felt fine. Though I was young and foolish, I instinctively knew I should get off the pill, which I did.

My doctor didn't understand and tried to talk me out of the decision. I have since learned that estrogen can trigger migraines.

At the time, I was taking an early formulation of the pill that contained 15 grams of estrogen.

Today, that concentration has been dramatically reduced to 20 – 50 micrograms.

(See: Pamela Verma Liao, MD and Janet Dollin, MD CM CCFP FCFP, "Half a Century of the Oral Contraceptive Pill: Historical Review and View to the Future," *Canadian Family Physician*, 2012 Dec: (58) 22.)

When I was growing up, many of us took up the common practice of smoking in high school or college. I have not smoked in more than forty-five years. I'm lucky to be here to write this book. At the time I took the pill, I also smoked, a deadly combination that can lead to strokes—a risk that still exists today with the reduced concentrations.

(See: Caitlin Carlton, Matthew Banks, and Sophia Sundararajan, "Oral Contraceptives and Ischemic Stroke Risk," *Stroke: AHA Journals*, 16 March 2018.)

After coming off the pill, I felt sick for more than a year. Everything bothered me. My nervous system seemed to be on high alert. Looking back, I think the culprit may have been flooding adrenaline and the first notable signs of MVPS. The weird, dream-like feelings did abate, but new problems emerged.

The Flip Side of the Birth Control Pill

During an annual checkup, my gynecologist noted polycystic ovary syndrome (PCOS), which can interfere with the development and release of eggs. Basically, I was not ovulating.

The doctor warned me that the longer I waited to treat the syndrome the less chance I would have of ever getting pregnant. I asked if taking birth control could have caused the PCOS. He said that could not be the case.

Which of us was crazy? Isn't the purpose of the birth control pill to stop ovulation?

I left the office with a referral to a fertility specialist who prescribed Clomid (clomiphene citrate). The drug stimulates ovulation by working on the pituitary gland to secrete more FSH and LH while, at the same time, stimulating the ovaries to secrete estrogen.

(See: "Clomiphene Citrate," *The Embryo Project Encyclopedia,* embryo.asu.edu.)

Birth control pills affect the pituitary gland to get the *opposite* results—stopping ovulation. I asked every doctor I saw if the birth control pills could have caused my infertility. I was always told no.

I have since found research that contradicts those assurances.

(See: D.R. Mishell Jr., O.A. Kletzky, P.F. Brenner, S. Roy, and J. Nicoloff, "The Effect of Contraceptive Steroids on Hypothalamic-Pituitary Function," *The American Journal of Obstetrics and Gynecology,* 1977 May 1(128) 1; and Kathy Chiapaikeo, "How Things Work: Birth Control Pills," *The Tartan,* 6 February 2006.)

At the time, the internet didn't exist for research. I was only twenty-three-years-old. All I had to depend on was my logical thinking and limited personal experience. Both screamed to me that the birth control pills caused the problem.

The Clomid worked. I was able to get pregnant. But I never trusted doctors again when it came to birth control pills, especially when they continued to recommend that I take them after the birth of my daughter. I never took the pill again.

Taking Clomid

Clomid changed my body. I felt flushed with hormones, but not in a good way.

The side effects included:

- hot flashes
- mood swings
- breast discomfort or tenderness
- nausea or vomiting
- bloating
- dizziness or light-headedness

Dizziness and headaches hit me the hardest, starting during a visit to the grocery store while I was on my first round of the drug.

The room began to spin. Feeling unbalanced, I left my cart, steadying myself as best I could on the walk to the car. Once seated, I waited until the feeling subsided enough that I felt safe to drive to the home of my husband's aunt.

I didn't want to be alone, because the episode had not fully resolved. I still felt a weird sensation.

I remember sitting in my in-law's home while she expressed her hope that the feeling would soon pass. She was very nice. Then the phone rang. While speaking with her friend, amusement replaced that supportive tone. She said she didn't know why I was there because I looked just fine.

Nothing could have been further from the truth. Looking back, I now know that the symptoms I felt were from a migraine aura triggered by adrenaline flooding my system. As awful as those feelings were, not knowing what was happening to me made it worse.

Reliving that episode, I think I might have walked down an aisle where fragrances or insecticides were shelved. Either could have triggered a migraine—they've done so many times since.

I believe that the heavy dose of hormones I was taking to help me get pregnant triggered the event and made me more susceptible to the chemicals.

After that incident, I was afraid to go anywhere alone because I did not know what had caused the dizzy, fainting feeling—or if it would happen again.

At one point I ended up in therapy for agoraphobia, known as the fear of being out in public. The therapy didn't help. My "agoraphobia" was resolved when my hormones came back into balance and I started to feel better.

How I Treat Migraines

Prevention means avoiding triggers, which for me include specific foods, odors or chemicals. Since avoidance isn't always possible or practical, I have developed strategies to help. For instance, if I think I'm having a food reaction, I dissolve two Alka-Seltzer Gold tablets (in the yellow box) in water and sip the drink. When I go out to dinner, I order club soda during the cocktail hour, a weaker form of the same neutralizer found in Alka-Seltzer Gold and keep it with me at the table during and after the meal.

Migraine First Aid Kit

I have several treatment options in my migraine first aid kit that can stop or reduce the episode. Many of these interventions are also effective for my arrhythmias.

The Homeopathic Remedy That Worked

A friend who suffered debilitating, painful migraines used nausea suppositories prescribed by her doctor that put her to sleep. When she awakened, the pain would be gone.

That gave me an idea. Since I respond well to homeopathic preparations, I turned to anti-nausea drops. The preparation helped— until the company stopped making the product. I panicked.

I purchased every last bottle I could find. When my supply ran out, I got creative, locating a homeopathic lab.

I wrote down the listed ingredients from the label on my bottle of anti-nausea drops and sent it to the lab to formulate the same preparation.

The ingredients listed on the bottle are:

- Aethusa cynapium (Fools Parsley) 4x
- Podophyllum peltatum (May Apple) 4x
- Anacardium orientale (making Nut) 6x
- Colchicum autumnale (meadow Saffron) 6x
- Ipecacuanha (Ipecac) 6x
- Iodium (Iodine) 12x

Other ingredients include purified water and 20% USP alcohol.

Disclaimer:
Please note that I am not advocating the use of this preparation. I list the ingredients and amounts here only as an illustration of a

homeopathic remedies that I have found to be helpful and how I was able to duplicate it when it was no longer available. It is an example of what anyone can do for themselves. Individuals are unique, and readers should conduct their own research into products or natural substances that are effective for their particular circumstances.

About Pain

Although I don't suffer from debilitating migraine pain, I do experience normal levels of headache pain and scary auras that can last for days. When I do have headache pain, I usually take extra-strength acetaminophen. I see no benefit in enduring pain when I can often break the cycle with a single dose of an over-the-counter painkiller.

Magnetic Head Bands and Sea Bands for Nausea

If I even think I feel a migraine coming on, I wear a magnetic headband and sea bands on my wrist, which are used for motion sickness. Then I take my homeopathic nausea drops and leave them under my tongue.

The headband can be tightened, which sometimes feels good in and of itself, but the magnets are supposed to help, too. Since I get auras, the sea bands help to counter that weird seasick feeling.

Weather changes can also trigger my migraines. Erratic and severe weather over the last few years have triggered variations in my symptoms. I feel the effect most strongly as the storm moves out.

I assume barometric pressure causes the reaction, but I have not been able to locate a specific treatment to counter the effect. The magnetic headband helps to a degree while I continue to search for a better method.

Magnesium

After swallowing the homeopathic nausea drops, I place liquid magnesium under my tongue. This sublingual method gets the mineral into my system more quickly, so I hold the magnesium under my tongue as long as possible

If I am out of the solution, I open magnesium capsules and stir the powder in warm water, which I then drink.

The goal is to get the mineral into my system as quickly as possible. Magnesium helps to relax the vessels and to stop the symptoms. If this doesn't help enough, I will contact my doctor and ask if I can get a magnesium injection.

Protein

Eating a piece of chicken, a hard-boiled egg, or some other form of quick protein can counteract hypoglycemia or low blood sugar.

The causes of hypoglycemia can be from not eating often enough, failing to consume adequate protein, and taking in too many refined carbohydrates.

When a person becomes hypoglycemic, the body releases adrenaline to help get stored glucose into the bloodstream quickly. Eating protein can help prevent that process. As noted earlier, adrenaline causes vasoconstriction which can trigger migraines.

Chocolate

A bite or two of 85% organic dark chocolate can also help. The tiny amount of sugar in this type of chocolate seems to work better for me than 100% chocolate. If that is all that is available, however, I dip the chocolate in organic honey.

Drink Water

In about one-third of migraine sufferers, dehydration triggers the event. Dehydration decreases the amount of blood in circulation. The blood thickens and flows with difficulty, making the heart beat harder and faster and potentially causing palpitations. Drinking water helps my migraines and is also good for GERD, arrhythmias and chest pain.

(See: "Top 10 Migraine Triggers and How to Deal with Them," *American Migraine Foundation*, 27 July 2017.)

Be Prepared

The faster I take these steps the sooner I feel better. Sometimes these measures stop the migraine in its tracks. I keep a large bottle of water next to my bed along with a plastic box that holds magnesium, homeopathic anti-nausea drops, acetaminophen, a magnetic headband and a set of the sea bands.

If I have the beginning of a migraine aura, I do not want to waste time trying to locate all the items that will help. That search wouldn't be easy under the influence of the weird feelings that accompany the aura.

As soon as I start this part of my protocol, I head for the kitchen to find some protein. Additionally, I use a new program, which I will describe in Chapter 16. My migraines are infrequent now, and I am more able to stop them early in the episode.

Chapter 11
Taking the Fear Out of Anxiety

Anxiety is a symptom, *not* a condition.

I have never had an anxiety disorder. Anxiety is a symptom, *not* a condition. Psychiatrists like to call the symptoms I've experienced "generalized anxiety." Some of my symptoms have even fit the diagnosis of agoraphobia and panic attacks.

Seeking therapy didn't help me. Finding a doctor and other professionals who treated the physical causes underlying my feeling of anxiety did.

Psychiatrists are fully licensed medical doctors. I would have assumed a professional with those credentials could have determined if medical issues affected my emotional state. Instead, they seem more inclined to prescribe some potent psychiatric drugs with lots of side effects to treat the symptoms. I don't find being labeled with a psychiatric or medical disorder based on my symptoms to be helpful.

Think about it this way. Should the flu be called a "fever and chills disorder"? The same can be said for anxiety. Should every experience of anxiety be labeled a "disorder"? In my opinion, that approach represents lazy medicine that overlooks the root cause of the problem.

My adrenaline and MVPS issues can cause anxiety. Knowing that information gives me options to treat the cause and calm things down. An anxiety diagnosis and accompanying prescription might also relieve the MVPS symptoms but ignores the adrenaline problem that causes them.

A Psychiatric Diagnosis

Psychiatric disorders are commonly treated with drugs that cover or lessen the symptoms. Those medications, if I were to take them, might make me feel better in the short run, but the symptoms will likely return when I stop taking the pills.

I'm not suggesting there's no benefit to feeling better, but for me, psychiatric drugs have the potential to cause more problems than they fix. Over the long term, some drugs in this class can cause serious cardiac issues and even death. MVPS does not. In addition, feeling anxious is not always a bad thing. Anxiety can be the body's way of alerting us to serious problems, like a heart attack.

Treatments for Anxiety Disorder

Conventional treatment for anxiety disorder consists of therapy and/or drugs. I like talk therapy with the right person for the right reasons. For example, after my divorce, I found counseling to be quite helpful. There were no drugs involved. The sessions were an excellent way to work out all the many changes happening in my life at the time.

A psychological approach to stopping the MVPS symptoms, however, does not work for me. I wish I could talk myself out of both the syndrome and the symptoms. I tried therapy for anxiety years ago before I knew about my adrenaline issues. The experience didn't help.

Drugs are also used to treat anxiety and panic disorders. Most everyone I've met who has been diagnosed with such a disorder takes a drug for the condition. The most common prescriptions are benzodiazepines such as Ativan®, Xanax® and Klonopin®. Valium also falls into this category but has some helpful nonpsychiatric uses.

For instance, Valium was effective for my urinary tract infection pain. As an older drug, the side effects of Valium are well-documented. I have had no problems with the medication, which also helped me again when a beta blocker left me with tremors and muscle twitches. Valium calmed my body during the many months I worked to recover. I don't reject all drugs, but I do prefer to use them carefully, for the right reasons, and as infrequently as possible.

Antidepressants and beta blockers are also prescribed for anxiety and panic. I don't take beta blockers for obvious reasons and would only consider the medications in a life-or-death scenario. I do know people who use beta blockers to cope with their fear of flying, a problem I addressed with the SOAR Program, which I will discuss in Chapter 16. Performers also use these drugs for stage fright.

The nervousness that I feel before acting in plays or speaking in public doesn't cause me any concern and actually helps improve my energy for the performance. Once on stage, I feel calmer but alert. At those times, the adrenaline in my body is a positive, normal thing.

Antidepressants come with a multitude of side effects. Stopping the use of these drugs can be difficult and even dangerous. (For more information, see: "Anxiety Medication," *Help Guide*, helpguide.org.)

Psychiatrist's Diagnostic and Statistical Manual

The Diagnostic and Statistical Manual of Mental Disorders (DSM) is considered the diagnostic bible for psychiatrists. The book lists psychiatric disorders and the symptoms used to describe those disorders.

Every few years, a group of psychiatrists gathers and vote to include certain groups of behaviors as psychiatric disorders. Through a simple vote, with no objective means of diagnosis, a new disorder becomes official.

If you have high blood pressure, your doctor can objectively measure that and give you a diagnosis of hypertension. If you have diabetes, your doctor can objectively measure your blood sugar and give you a diagnosis of diabetes. Psychiatric disorders are subjective. There are no objective tests to prove that the condition exists. To further complicate treatment, some emotional behaviors can be symptoms of other medical problems.

(For more information, see: Steven T. Dorsey, MD, "Medical Conditions that Mimic Psychiatric Disease: A Systematic Approach for Evaluation of Patients Who Present with Psychiatric Symptomatology," *Relias Media*, 22 September 2002.)

The DSM Listing for Anxiety

The DSM-5™ lists the following diagnostic criteria for generalized anxiety disorder:

1. Excessive anxiety and worry occurring more days than not for at least six months.
2. The individual finds it difficult to control the worry.
3. The anxiety and worry are associated with three (or more) of the following six symptoms (with at least some symptoms having been present for more days than not for the past six months). *
4. Restlessness, feeling keyed up or on edge.
5. Being easily fatigued.
6. Difficulty concentrating or mind going blank.
7. Irritability.
8. Muscle tension.
9. Sleep disturbance (difficulty falling or staying asleep, or restless, unsatisfying sleep).
10. The anxiety, worry, or physical symptoms cause clinically significant distress or impairment in social, occupational, or other important areas of functioning.

11. The disturbance is not attributable to the physiological effects of a substance (e.g., a drug of abuse, a medication) or another medical condition (e.g., hyperthyroidism).
12. The disturbance is not better explained by another medical disorder.
   Note: Only one item is required in children.

Anxiety—A Dubious Diagnosis

These symptoms and their duration are used to diagnose people considered to have an anxiety disorder. My MVPS symptoms can fit nicely in that list. I'm sure some doctors I have seen would have liked to label me with this dubious disorder, but they may have overlooked the last entry on the DMS list: "The disturbance is not better explained by another medical disorder."

For me, anxiety and panic most often occur when adrenaline is released on its own. That is when nothing I have done would trigger that release. My adrenals malfunction and release the hormone without external or emotional provocation. When I am upset, I feel like I am getting a double dose of adrenaline.

No one seems to consider that I may have a dysfunction of the autonomic nervous system. Identifying that process and addressing it makes more sense to me than trying to fit me into the Diagnostic Criteria of Generalized Anxiety Disorder and handing me a prescription for antianxiety medication with all the related side effects.

What My Previous Doctors Could Learn from Dr. Oz

Several years ago, while watching television, I heard Dr. Oz say that MVP (without the syndrome) was a leading cause of panic attacks. He explained that the snapping back of the prolapsed valve at closure produces vibrations that shake the back wall of the heart, stimulating nerves in that region. In that moment the person feels panic as if they were being attacked.

The explanation sounded like Physiology 101. Did my previous doctors skip that day of medical school? Were they asleep in their seats? Miss the question on the exam?

These same doctors could hear the click and read the echocardiogram, but no one explained what was happening to me as clearly as a doctor on television. That segment is available on Dr. Oz's website for any physician looking to expand their knowledge of MVP.

(See: "Panic Problems: Mitral Valve Prolapse," *Oz*, doctoroz.com.)

Misinformation, however, can and does grow in the medical profession. In a research study published in 2008, "Does the Association Between Mitral Valve Prolapse and Panic Disorder Really Exist?," the authors conclude:

"Published results are insufficient to definitely establish or to exclude an association between MVP and panic disorder. If any relationship does actually exist, it could be said to be infrequent and mainly occur in subjects with minor variants of MVP. To clarify this intriguing issue, future studies should mainly focus on the observed methodological biases and particularly should use the current criteria for MVP as the standard for evaluation."

(See: Alaor Santos Filho, M.D., Benedito C. Maciel, M.D., Ph.D., and José Alexandre Crippa, M.D., Ph.D., et al, "Does the Association Between Mitral Valve Prolapse and Panic Disorder Really Exist?" *Primary Care Companion to The Journal of Clinical Psychiatry,* 2008 [10] 1.)

The authors uncovered nothing conclusive when they could have reviewed the basic physiology of a floppy valve. To me, their research, which helped no one, was a waste of time.

Panic Attacks

The DSM lists panic attacks as a separate disorder described as a sudden, intense fear without danger or cause. A person should have at least four of the listed symptoms to receive a diagnosis. During an MVPS flare-up, I experience everything on the list. A panic attack, characterized by a sense of impending doom or danger, also signals a heart attack.

The following list of panic attack symptoms includes asterisks indicating which sensations also signal a cardiac event:

- Abdominal cramping
- Chest pain*
- Chills
- Dizziness*
- Light-headedness or faintness*
- Fear of loss of control or death
- Feeling of unreality or detachment
- Headache
- Hot flashes
- Nausea*
- Numbness or tingling sensation
- Rapid, racing or pounding heart rate*
- Sense of impending doom or danger*
- Shortness of breath or tightness in your throat*
- Sweating*
- Trembling or shaking.*

Other medical conditions also cause anxiety or can be indicated by anxiety.

Panic and Anxiety Can Be Caused by or Can Indicate a Medical Issue

These include, but may not be limited to:

- Heart disease
- Diabetes
- Thyroid problems, such as hyperthyroidism
- Respiratory disorders, such as chronic obstructive pulmonary disease and asthma
- Withdrawal from alcohol, antianxiety medications or other medications
- Chronic pain or irritable bowel syndrome
- Rare tumors that produce certain fight-or-flight hormones
- A side effect of certain medications

(See: "Anxiety Disorders," *Mayo Clinic*, mayoclinic.org.)

Other Nonpsychiatric Causes of Anxiety and Panic Attacks: Treatment or Prevention

Obviously, as per Dr. Oz's explanation, a floppy mitral valve belongs on this list. People can't prevent the stimulation of the nerves at the back of the heart, but they can reduce the effect.

When I get that anxious or panicky feeling out of the blue, I don't panic over the panic. Simply knowing what causes the sensation allows me not to react with fear which can result in flooding my system with even more stress hormones.

Panic Causes More Panic: The Domino Effect and How to Stop It

Captain Tom Bunn, the author of *Panic Free: The 10-Day Program to End Panic, Anxiety, and Claustrophobia*, calls this the domino effect, which, if allowed to run unchecked, will cause a full-blown panic attack. He has an effective retraining system that he likens to a strand of pearls.

The knots between the individual pearls on a strand prevent all the beads from falling when the string breaks. His system separates or neutralizes each element of a panic attack so that no matter where the panic starts that is also where it stops. (Later in this chapter and Chapter 16, I will discuss Bunn's system at greater length.)

Hypoglycemia

One doctor I know maintains that unless proven otherwise hypoglycemia or low blood sugar causes anxiety or panic attacks. When I reviewed this condition, it made perfect sense.

Hypoglycemia results from:

- Inadequate protein consumption
- Infrequent meals
- Eating foods high in sugar

When a person becomes hypoglycemic, the body releases adrenaline to help get stored glucose into the bloodstream quickly.

When that happens, I'm right back to dealing with the effects of adrenaline, the chemical underlying most of my MVPS symptoms—and the one that can cause a feeling of anxiety.

In addition to the direct effect of adrenaline, some of the symptoms of low blood sugar can make the adrenaline reaction worse. These include:

- Hunger
- Dizziness
- Fatigue
- Sleepiness
- General weakness

- Heart palpitations
- Nervousness
- Shakiness
- Sweating
- Anxiety

Eating several small meals a day, including protein and avoiding sugar, helps me to prevent episodes of hypoglycemia.

Low Magnesium

Low magnesium levels also can make me feel mildly driven and anxious. As "nature's valium," the calming effect of magnesium can increase focus and concentration.

Histamine

During an allergic reaction, the body releases histamine, which it then tries to reduce by releasing adrenaline. Avoiding allergens or treating them as soon as possible can help prevent the flooding of adrenaline into the system.

The Limbic System

The limbic system, sometimes referred to as the body's "first responder," determines our level of safety.

It reacts to both perceived and real threats, sending survival messages to the rest of the body to take action. Analyzing and filtering incoming stimuli, the limbic system assigns a level of importance to each potential threat and remembers that in order to protect us in the future.

For example, if you touch a hot stove and get burned, the limbic system will help you remember not to do it again.

Sometimes, however, the limbic system can become hypersensitive to a painful or scary experience, causing a recurring over firing of protective chemicals such as adrenaline to any future situations that are similar. Programs exist to counteract this sequence. See: "Dynamic Neural Retraining System" at retrainingthebrain.com.

(For more information on the stress response, see, "Understanding the Stress Response," *Harvard Health Publishing: Harvard Medical School*, health.harvard.edu.)

I believe that in an effort to protect me, my limbic system has caused most of my MVPS-related anxiety. The first time this occurred, as I explained in a previous chapter, I was in my early twenties when I suffered a panic attack in the grocery store. At the time, I was taking the fertility drug Clomid.

Now I understand that I was experiencing an aura triggered by the drug, which elevates the risk for migraines. I felt weak, dizzy, shaky and unsteady. After that occurred, whenever I attempted to go into stores, I felt the same panicked feeling.

I believe this was my limbic system trying to warn me of the danger I felt the first time I had that negative experience.

That reaction stopped me from going in at all or forced me to flee. I was diagnosed with agoraphobia (the fear of public places), but therapy didn't help.

Later, however, as the effects of the drug wore off, my constant fears and feelings of anxiety stopped.

The brain's protective reaction to that traumatic event made me think about my reactions to MVPS symptoms. Those first episodes of chest pain or stroke-like migraine headaches imprinted a memory of danger in my brain. When those symptoms happened again, my limbic system jumped into survival mode.

As adrenaline triggered a fight-or-flight response, my brain's accelerated survival instinct made me believe that the symptoms were serious each time. My brain may well have been alerting me to a danger that didn't exist. This is the premise of an effective therapy that helps people recover from chronic illnesses. More on this in Chapter 16.

My research reveals many physiological processes that cause anxiety. This is why I prefer to find the underlying physical cause of what I am feeling rather than accept both a psychiatric diagnosis and an antianxiety drug.

I never think of anxiety as a psychiatric disorder. With MVPS alone, there are many symptoms that can cause a feeling of anxiety. When I hear someone is suffering from anxiety, I wonder what medical condition is not being diagnosed or treated.

The Problem with Breathing Techniques

I have never had much success using breathing techniques. I thought it was because I wasn't doing it correctly. I tried the most common system referred to as the 4-7-8 breathing method. This system teaches a cycle of breathing that starts with inhaling through the nose for a count of four and then holding it for a count of seven. Once done, the person should completely exhale through the mouth for a count of eight. I even bought a biofeedback device that claims to help reduce stress by using a specific breathing pattern.

The graph on the screen showed me when to inhale and how long to hold my breath before exhaling.

I used it for several months but never felt like I got much benefit. I do know that slowing my breathing in general can be helpful but nothing more specific than that. Then I read an article by Captain Bunn on how to turn on the parasympathetic system which can help counter the effects of the "fight or flight" response.

The article, "The Part of the Brain That Stops Anxiety and How to Use It," *Psychology Today*, February 5, 2021, was very helpful and revealed the limits of using breathing techniques to calm the sympathetic system. Bunn explains in the article, "Though exhaling activates the parasympathetic system, inhaling deactivates it. It's like opening and closing your parapluie (umbrella) repeatedly in a rainstorm as a way to stay dry."

Instead of using breathing techniques, I now use the techniques explained by Captain Bunn in his book, *Panic Free: The 10-Day Program to End Panic, Anxiety, and Claustrophobia, with* better results. Some of Bunn's techniques are explained in this chapter beginning with his recommended method for self-calming.

A Method for Self-Calming
How To Override the Sympathetic Nervous System

Dr. Stephen Porges, a neurologist and researcher, discovered a method that people can use to calm themselves, even when alone. Here's how it works. According to Dr. Porges, we are genetically programmed to be calmed by the "face, voice quality, and body language/touch" of a person who does not judge us but accepts us. Being with this person can make us feel calm and safe. Porges explains that it is an unconscious process where calming signals are sent and received between these two people. It is this exchange that activates the parasympathetic system which then counters and can override the sympathetic system that controls the fight-or-flight response. This calming can occur even if adrenaline is being released and can signal the body to stop releasing it. We can do this when we are alone by visualizing the "calming" person.

More on this method and Dr. Porges can be found in two excellent articles by Captain Tom Bunn, author of the book *Panic Free: The 10-Day Program to End Panic, Anxiety, and Claustrophobia*. Captain Bunn also developed the SOAR Program for nervous flyers that worked so well for me and is discussed in more detail in Chapter 16.

(Captain Tom Bunn, L.C.S.W., "How To Stop A Panic Attack and Keep It From Happening Again," Psychology Today, June 15, 2020.)

(Captain Tom Bunn, L.C.S.W., "The Psychological Discovery That Can Keep You Calm During This Crisis." *Medium.com*, July 20, 2020.

(See the book by Dr. Porges, *Polyvagal Safety: Attachment, Communication, Self-Regulation*.)

(See an article by Dr. Porges, "The Anatomy of Calm," Psychology Today, September 7, 2021)

The Three-Button Exercise to Help Relieve Stress

The following information is from the book *Panic Free* by Tom Bunn with permission from the author.

This is the exercise to use if you notice you are stressed about something. Remember a person with whom you've felt your guard let down. The signals that cause your guard to let down are transmitted by the person's face, their voice, and their touch. I want you to imagine buttons you can press to calm yourself.

Imagine your friend has pasted a sticker on their forehead bearing a picture of a button with the number 1 on it. Another sticker, showing button number 2, is pasted on their chin. A third sticker, with button number 3, is pasted on the back of their hand. Now imagine feeling alarmed.

Imagine putting your finger on the button 1 sticker on their forehead and then releasing it. Their face comes clearly to mind. You see the softness in their eyes. It feels good.

Imagine putting your finger on the button 2 sticker. As you release it, the person's lips begin to move, and you hear them greet you in a special way. You may notice that the quality of their voice calms you deep inside.

Imagine touching the button 3 sticker on the back of their hand. When you release the button, the person lifts their hand and gives you a reassuring touch or a hug —whatever gesture is appropriate in your relationship with this person. You may notice calming stillness rest on you.

Linking the Three Button Exercise to the Actual Experience that Causes Anxiety

You can calm yourself by pressing the buttons any time you wish. But we want to set up calming that works automatically.

To establish automatic attenuation (reduction of the anxiety), intentionally remember feeling alarmed and then:

- Press button 1.
- Remember the feeling again; press button 2.
- Bring the feeling to mind again; press button 3.

Linking the Three Button Exercise to the Symptoms of Anxiety

Now we'll fine-tune the exercise with steps that link the three buttons to the specific things you feel when highly aroused or anxious.

Remember feeling your heart beat faster. Imagine pressing button 1 to bring to mind the memory of the person's calming face. This establishes a visual link between being aroused and then calmed by the softness of their face and gaze.

As you remember feeling your heart beat faster, imagine you are pressing button 2 to hear a conversation you and your friend might have about that feeling. This links your increased heart rate to calming signals in your friend's voice.

As you remember feeling your heart beat faster, pretend you are pressing button 3 to feel your friend's reassuring touch. This establishes a link between arousal and calming touch.

Remember feeling your breathing get faster. Pressing button 1 brings to mind your friend's calming face to establish a visual link to that sensation.

Next, establish a vocal link between rapid breathing and your friend's calming voice by pressing button 2. Have a pretend conversation with your friend about your rapid breathing.

As you notice your breathing, press button 3 and imagine the reassuring touch of your friend's hand.

Recall starting to feel tense. Press button 1 as soon as you feel tension, bringing your friend's face to mind.

Again, as you start to feel tense, press button 2 and imagine your friend is saying something to you.

As soon you begin to feel tense, use button 3 to remember feeling your friend's calming touch.

Use The Three Button Exercise Using Cartoon Characters

Now, as an expcriment, try a variation of the exercise using cartoon characters. This can reduce the anxiety associated with the exercise. We don't take it seriously when cartoon characters are distressed, because we know it will all work out in the end. Try it and see which version you prefer.

Imagine the cartoon character's heart beat faster. Press button 1 and imagine that your friend is holding the cartoon by their face. As you see your friend's face and the cartoon, notice your friend's eyes.

Imagine the cartoon character feeling their heart beat faster. Imagine you are pressing button 2 to hear a conversation you and your friend might have about the cartoon character's experience of that feeling.

As you look at the cartoon with your friend, pretend you are pressing button 3 to feel your friend's reassuring touch.

Imagine the cartoon character's breathing getting faster. Press button 1 and imagine your friend is holding the cartoon by their face to establish a visual link.

Next, establish a vocal link between rapid breathing and your friend's calming voice by pressing button 2. Imagine a conversation with your friend about the cartoon character's rapid breathing.

As you talk about the cartoon character's rapid breathing, press button 3 and imagine the touch of your friend's hand.

Think of a cartoon character feeling tense. Press button 1. Bring your friend's face to mind. Imagine the cartoon by your friend's face.

Press button 2 and imagine you and your friend are talking about the cartoon character's tension.

As you and your friend have that conversation, use button 3 to bring to mind the feeling of your friend's calming touch.

A Note from Joan Anderson

The exercises, explained above by Captain Bunn, have worked exceptionally well for me in many situations including flying which is why I was pleased, that, with Bunn's permission, I could share them in this book. The training automatically kicks in when I am in a stressful situation without me thinking about it. Being calm in these situations now feels natural to me. I learned much from his book, "Panic Free" but also from the videos included in the SOAR program for fearful flyers that he developed. In some of the videos, Bunn walks clients through the exercises as a demonstration which helped me go through the steps more effectively on my own.

Thinking Fast or Slow Matters

"Most people with a fear of flying and anxiety are pretty much locked into thinking fast," explained Captain Tom Bunn in one of his weekly newsletters for people like me who took his SOAR course that addressed my fear of flying. Over the years since I finished the course and became a comfortable flyer as a result, he has continued to update me and other SOAR participants with more information to help relieve anxiety. I look forward to reading his updates every Wednesday. In his last newsletter before I wrote this section, he explained two systems of thinking—fast and slow—and the effect they can have on provoking or relieving anxiety. With Bunn's permission, I will share some of his article.

In his newsletter, Bunn discusses fast and slow thinking, a concept developed by Nobel Prize Winner Daniel Kahneman in his book *Thinking Fast and Slow*. Kahneman contends that fast thinking is intuitive and emotional and slow thinking is more deliberative and more logical. I write about this concept in Chapter 1 in the section "Who's in Control, Me or My Lizard Brain?" In his newsletter, Bunn describes certain techniques that can help us tap into the benefits of slow thinking and how it can prevent or relieve anxiety and fear often caused by fast (reactive) thinking.

Bunn explained that fast thinkers with anxiety are often reluctant to slow down their thinking and review the subject because they worry that just the act of thinking about it will provoke more anxiety. Yet it is this slow, deliberate thinking that allows a person to review, critique and oftentimes resolve their concerns, which can reduce the anxiety. Using slow thinking can be helpful for patients. Bunn explained that thinking slow and deliberately about medical issues rather than having a knee-jerk reaction can help patients make calmer, more deliberate decisions.

Dr. Stephen Porges and the Social Engagement System

During my discussions with Captain Tom Bunn on the nervous system, he emailed me the following information on how Dr. Stephen Porges discovered how the calming system works. It is informal but very interesting so, with Bunn's permission, I thought I would share it in this book.

Dr. Porges stumbled on this discovery—that a completely accepting person tends to send us unconscious signals that calm us—when he was doing research on the vagus nerve, the nerve that when stimulated slows our heart rate and relaxes our gut. This is the opposite of what the sympathetic nervous system—the system that revs us up—does.

When the amygdala picks up a possible threat (that may be giving it too much credit, as it reacts to any unexpected change as a possible threat), it releases stress hormones. The stress hormones cause the sympathetic nervous system to sound the alarm that there may be a threat, and in case the threat is real, it prepares us for action.

It increases our heart rate and breathing rate. It borrows the blood supply to the digestive system and reroutes it to the muscles, so we are better able to run or fight. (That explains why, if stress persists, we have digestive problems.)

The parasympathetic nervous system does the opposite. If there is evidence that we are safe, the parasympathetic overrides the sympathetic. It reverses the increased heart rate. It relaxes the gut. And the evidence that we are safe is right there in the face of a friend, right there in the quality of their voice, and right there in their touch.

Since the amygdala fires off every time we encounter a new person, our ability to pick up signals from their face, voice, and body language keeps us from going automatically into fighting them or fleeing from them or freezing like a deer in the headlights. The way he stumbled on this is interesting. He had a research subject hooked up to equipment that could instantly pick up changes in heart rate. He was surprised to see that when a friend of the person connected to his equipment walked by their heart rate went dramatically down.

That was the beginning of what he now calls the "Social Engagement System," the system that apparently makes human relatedness and cooperation possible through feelings of security when we unconsciously pick up safety signals from others.

Read more on how to activate your parasympathetic system in the Forward, written by Bunn.

Chapter 12
Just Because You Feel Depressed
Doesn't Mean You Have Depression
Handling the Symptom Without Antidepressants

IMPORTANT

No one should ever rapidly discontinue the use of antidepressants. Stopping an antidepressant should always be done slowly and under the supervision of a knowledgeable doctor.

Disclaimer

If you are in crisis or having suicidal thoughts, immediately call your doctor, 911, or the National Suicide Prevention Lifeline at 1-800-273-TALK (8255) to speak with a trained counselor. If you are located outside the United States, call your local emergency line immediately.

How MVPS Symptoms Can Make Me Feel Sad

When my MVPS symptoms flared and practically stopped me in my tracks, I felt immense sadness. I had other plans for my life. I certainly didn't want to spend my time and precious energy fighting MVPS.

I can understand why anyone would feel depressed trying to live a normal life with MVPS. Still, I contend that reaction should not receive a psychiatric diagnosis, nor do I think an antidepressant would help the actual problem or even be an effective coping strategy. After the birth of my second child, I took an antidepressant for constant right-side abdominal pain, which was described to me as a symptom of postpartum depression. While I didn't believe that to be true, the doctors weren't offering other options, so I briefly went along. The drug didn't help the pain, which turned out to be my appendix. Surgery, not an antidepressant, fixed the problem.

Causes of My Depressed Feelings

I have had some extended periods of feeling down or depressed, but I didn't even consider going to a psychiatrist. I always take my symptoms to a medical doctor to search for the real root of the problem.

Some conditions that can cause a feeling of depression for me include:

- Low hormone levels after a hysterectomy.
- Low thyroid levels after menopause.
- Low vitamin B levels.
- Depleted magnesium levels.
- A difficult marriage.

All of the first four on the list were medically addressed without resorting to antidepressants, and a divorce solved the fifth one.

Another Look at Magnesium

An article from the Cleveland Clinic, "Depression & Heart Disease," by Leo Pozuelo, MD, asserts that depression can increase the risk of cardiac disease for those with underlying cardiac issues. Additionally, depression can increase the risk of an adverse cardiac event like a heart attack or blood clots—a connection I have seen cited on other medical websites.

But this does not comport with research presented at Acute Cardiovascular Care 2018, a European Society of Cardiology congress in Milan, Italy. During those proceedings, data presented found heart attack patients prescribed antidepressants have lower one-year survival rates. ("Heart Attack Patients Prescribed Antidepressants Have Worse One-Year Survival," *European Society of Cardiology*, 3 March 2018.)

By focusing on depression as a cause, are doctors overlooking depression as a possible symptom of magnesium deficiency? Could untreated low magnesium cause the adverse cardiac events?

A 2013 article in *Medical News Today* by Kelly Fizgerald bears out the connection between magnesium levels and cardiac risk:

"The fact that low levels of magnesium are associated with all the risk factors and symptoms of heart disease, hypertension, diabetes, high cholesterol, heart arrhythmia, angina and heart attack can no longer be ignored; the evidence is much too compelling." (See: Kelly Fitzgerald, "Low Magnesium Linked to Heart Disease," *Medical News Today*, 2 February 2013.)

Additionally, an article by Lawrence K. Altman that appeared in *The New York Times* on June 28, 1992, asserted that magnesium is an effective treatment for a heart attack survivor to prevent a second attack.

(See: Lawrence K. Altman, "A Study Finds Magnesium Cut Deaths by Heart Attack," *The New York Times*, 28 June 1992. Please note that web access to this article may require a subscription to *The New York Times* as per the newspaper's online access policy.)

An antidepressant, with all its serious side effects, does nothing for a magnesium deficiency, which puts a person at a higher risk of a heart attack. This raises a clear question. Does depression increase the risk of a heart attack or does low magnesium cause both the depression and the heart attack?

Allergies

Yes, allergies can cause depression. Both depression and allergies can run in families. Some references in the medical literature suggest that it is the inflammation from the allergy that alters brain chemistry, causing the depression.

(See: Maria Cohut, PhD, "Are Allergies Linked to Anxiety and Depression?" *Medical News Today*, 29 May 2019.)

Antidepressants Were Actually Antihistamines

The first antidepressants produced were formulated from antihistamines. That should be a big clue that there is a real association between the two problems. These antidepressants are the tricyclic antidepressants such as:

- Tofranil
- Norpramin
- Anafranil
- Elavil
- Pamelor
- Sinequan
- Surmontil

Tricyclic antidepressants are potent antihistamines, which may explain their effectiveness for depression. (Elliott Richelson, M.D., "Pharmacology of Antidepressants—Characteristics of the Ideal Drug," *Mayo Clinic Proceedings,* 1 November 1994.)

(For more information, see: Dr. Mary Ann Block, *Just Because You're Depressed Doesn't Mean You Have Depression*, 28 April 2008.)

If I felt depressed, I would want a doctor to evaluate me for allergies and, if needed, treat them.

Most Common Medical Issues That Can Cause the Feeling of Depression

Dr. Block's book explains all the reasons why I don't believe in the depression diagnosis or look to antidepressants for treatment. The new antidepressants have serious side effects that are, in my estimation, not worth the risk.

If antidepressants were effective, why are drug companies advertising additional drugs to boost those very medications?

Dr. Block explains the six most common causes of the feeling of depression that she sees in her practice. They are:

- Thyroid problems
- Hormone deficiencies
- Magnesium and other nutritional deficiencies
- Allergies
- Prescription drug side effects
- A personal loss or other normal life cycle experience.

Problems with Antidepressants

In addition to the many news reports linking antidepressants to suicidal behavior, there are other side effects I find just plain scary. These include:

- Depression
  (Yes, antidepressants can also cause depression!)
- Heart failure
- Heart attack
- Atrial fibrillation
- Stroke
- Shock
- Thrombosis
- Ventricular arrhythmia and fibrillation

- Hemorrhage
- Coma
- Delusions
- Abnormal EEG
- Hypertension
- Angina pectoris
- Agitation
- Sleep disorders
- Apathy
- Ataxia
- Hallucinations
- Hostility
- Paranoid reactions
- Personality disorders
- Psychosis
- Vertigo
- Antisocial behavior
- Stupor

This is why I always research the potential side effects of prescribed medication. I have found doctors to be too quick to prescribe drugs. In my experience, most depression or sadness could be a natural response to a life situation not a medical condition. Such a symptom needs more attention. I do not believe it needs to be masked by a drug.

A Word About Normal Sadness

There are times when sadness is a normal response to a life event. If such feelings are treated too quickly, a person might lose the opportunity to use depression as a way to identify and deal with difficult problems.

For example, if someone you love dies or you suffer another kind of loss, sadness is expected. To give a grieving person an antidepressant will only prevent that person from feeling sad, cutting them off from processing their grief.

Many professionals agree. Writing for *Psychology Today* (4 March 2012), Alex Lickerman, MD, argues in "The Benefit of Sadness" that there are valid reasons to avoid such a situation. Suppressing unpleasant feelings because we're afraid of pain typically leads to greater pain in the future.

In "Why Bad Moods Are Good for You: The Surprising Benefits of Sadness," (ABC News Australia, 15 May 2017) Joseph Paul Forgas writes that bad moods are an essential part of the normal range of moods we regularly experience.

Grieving my losses helps me come to terms with them, and through that process, it helps me move on. However, some people may need more help. We are not all the same, nor do we all deal with the same issues.

Anyone in crisis or having suicidal thoughts should call their doctor, 911, or the National Suicide Prevention Lifeline at 1-800-273-TALK (8255) to speak to a trained counselor. If located outside the United States, call a local emergency line immediately

Chapter 13
Why I Feel It in My Gut and
How I Treat IBS, GERD and Gastritis

Irritable bowel syndrome is a functional problem of the gut, not a disease. The medical system sometimes calls this functional bowel disorders (FBD), a term that describes a problem with the function of the stomach and bowels. There is, however, no disease or abnormality as would be present in a condition like Crohn's disease, which can also cause inflammation of the skin, eyes, joints, liver or bile ducts.

A colonoscopy showed that my colon looked fine even though two days earlier I was doubled over with an IBS attack. My GI doctor offered no further information except that he'd never seen anyone so well cleaned out than I was. Really? Extremely painful cramps, that empty my colon, is a common occurrence with an IBS flare-up. I didn't expect that to be considered a medical upside.

The bottom line, however, is that even after that excruciating episode of an IBS attack, my colon looked healthy, and I was fine. That reassured me that what I have is a functional problem, not a physical one.

There are four types of IBS. (I have the first.)

- Pain and Cramping
- Diarrhea
- Constipation
- Alternating Constipation and Diarrhea

My research for this book uncovered the fact that anxiety and depression are now considered to be IBS symptoms. Frankly, I'm starting to take this personally.

It's bad enough that my MVPS symptoms flag me as a good target for antidepressant and antianxiety drugs. Now IBS apparently reinforces that judgment. I can be feeling perfectly calm and happy before I have an IBS attack—and go right back to being calm and happy when it's over.

Although I don't take psychiatric drugs, I do take a very effective medication when I feel the onset of cramps, which can almost immediately prevent or lessen the severity of the attack.

How I Found the Best Medication for My Type of IBS

In the dead of the night when the worst stomach pain I'd ever experienced woke me from a deep sleep, I didn't know if I could tolerate the severe cramping and unproductive pain. I grabbed the only drug given to me for my IBS, paregoric, a narcotic used for diarrhea in children and adults. In all the years I used it, it had never helped to stop or even decrease the IBS pain. At best, I could hope to feel groggy, and that usually occurred after the attack was over when I didn't need it. But no doctor had ever recommended anything else.

That episode was actually a colon bleed. When I stopped passing blood, I was left shaking and almost in shock. At the emergency room, they took my condition seriously, telling me that blood in the colon can be very painful. No kidding. By that time, however, the bleeding and most of the pain had stopped.

The ER doctor ordered an injection of Bentyl for me. Everything immediately calmed down. They sent me to a room where I let the drug lull me off to sleep.

I was beginning to heal. Later a colonoscopy found the cause of the bleed—mild irritation.

It never occurred to me that the enteric aspirin, also known as a "safety aspirin," I took daily for a painful twisted ankle would cause a bleed. I was wrong. My doctor identified the aspirin as the culprit.

Enteric aspirin, which is coated to prevent dissolution in the upper stomach, instead dissolves in the lower colon where it causes irritation. The aspirin further exacerbated the bleeding by interfering with blood clotting. Medical professionals commonly recommend taking an aspirin daily or at the first sign of a heart attack to prevent or break up a blood clot that may be the cause of a blockage to the heart.

(For more information, see the staff article: "Daily Aspirin Therapy: Understand the Benefits and Risks," *Mayo Clinic*, mayoclinic.org.)

The Three Things I Learned About IBS

First, I learned to take Tylenol, not aspirin, for pain or inflammation. I will occasionally take baby aspirin and carry them with me should I have a cardiac event. I have also been given baby aspirin in the ER for chest pain. This limited use doesn't cause any problems.

Second, I have a small, tortuous colon. Food passes through the winding, twisting, looping passage with great difficulty. It's little wonder my colon overreacts with strong contractions that turn into painful spasms. Before my first colonoscopy, my GI doctor reviewed my history and chose to use a pediatric scope. It would appear that my anatomy, not anxiety or depression, causes my IBS.

When I left the hospital after the bleed, the GI doctor prescribed Levsin for my IBS, which I did take for several weeks. My colon was so irritated that I was having severe cramps almost every day, which the drug didn't stop. Levsin was a newer drug at that time, and everyone seemed to be using it, but it was doing nothing for me.

Then I remembered that wonderful injection in the ER that calmed all my symptoms. I looked up Bentyl (dicyclomine) in the PDR:

"Dicyclomine is used to treat irritable bowel syndrome. It helps to reduce the symptoms of stomach and intestinal cramping. It works by slowing the natural movements of the gut and by relaxing the

muscles in the stomach and intestines. Class of drugs: anticholinergics/antispasmodics."

Unlike Levsin, which was a new, popular drug at the time, Bentyl had been used for years. I wanted it!

My GI doctor insisted I stay on Levsin. I called my primary care doctor and asked for Bentyl, which he prescribed in pill form, which didn't work quickly enough to halt an attack. Turning next to my pharmacist, I discovered Bentyl also comes in liquid form. That made more sense to me. My doctor changed the prescription, and just as I hoped it would, the liquid worked faster and better. Bentyl, in its liquid form, is now my drug of choice for IBS.

I carry the medication in a bottle with a dropper. At the first twinge of pain, I swallow a partial dose of the medication. Then I put drops under my tongue, a sublingual dose. Sublingual absorption is more efficient and works faster than an oral dose because the tiny blood vessels in the mouth allow the drug to be absorbed directly into the bloodstream without going through the digestive system.

How Close I Came to Danger

Because I don't have diarrhea as a major aspect of my IBS, I dodged a medical bullet. My doctor mentioned a new drug to me, Lotronex, that was for people with IBS with diarrhea. Because of my infrequent episodes of loose bowels, he thought I might try it to see if it would help. I declined.

Later when I looked up Lotronex, I learned the drug had been removed from the market due to reports of serious complications. "Alosetron hydrochloride (Lotronex), a prescription drug manufactured by GlaxoWellcome, and used to treat irritable bowel syndrome in women, has been withdrawn after reports of serious complications."

In the cases of women who took Lotronex cited in the report I read, there were:

- 70 cases of serious adverse events
- 49 cases of ischemic (restricting blood flow) colitis
- 21 cases of severe constipation
- 34 who were admitted to the hospital without surgery
- 10 who required surgical procedures
- 3 deaths
- 2 additional reports of death from other complications

(See: F. Charatan, "Drug for Irritable Bowel Syndrome Taken Off the Market," *British Medical Journal*, 2000 Dec 9;321[7274]:1429.)

What I Learn Over and Over Again

- Trust my body and research all drugs before using them.
- New drugs are not always better or safer, just highly marketed.
- Check for and review old, well-established drugs with a known history of side effects and efficacy.
- Don't follow doctor's orders if they don't make sense. Discuss other options with him or her instead.

Bentyl Has Side Effects Too

Bentyl comes with a slew of side effects, but none have been a problem for me. Unlike many new drugs, the side effects of old drugs like Bentyl have been well documented. I know what the side-effects are so I can identify them should I experience any of them. Also, I do not take the drug regularly which can increase the potential of a side effect. I only take Bentyl when I feel an attack coming on. I have been told to take the medication four times a day to prevent an IBS attack, but I prefer to use drugs only as needed. I try to prevent attacks by using more natural methods.

How I Help Prevent IBS Attacks

My food sensitivities can cause an IBS attack, so I try to avoid eating those items. Sometimes eating too much roughage can trigger an attack. I love salads and other raw fruits and vegetables, but I have to eat them sparingly. When I do have an attack caused by a food sensitivity, there are treatments I use to stop or prevent the reaction.

Alka Seltzer Gold

Alka Seltzer Gold, which is packed in an orange box and contains no aspirin, can sometimes stop or ease a food sensitivity reaction. I carry a two-pack in my purse along with Bentyl. I dissolve the Alka Seltzer tablet in a cup of water and sip the mixture.

Club soda can be used as a milder neutralizer. The beverage is easy to find, especially in restaurants that serve mixed drinks. I also have allergy drops but cannot carry them with me because they require refrigeration. Sometimes I will take my allergy drops before I leave the house to go out for a meal.

Quercetin

Quercetin acts like an antihistamine and an anti-inflammatory. It can stop a variety of allergic reactions by helping to stabilize mast cells, which release histamine and are the body's first line of defense against invaders. Mast cells, however, are also thought to cause chronic inflammation, which is why mast cell inhibitors like Quercetin are often used as a treatment.

[See: Mirjam Urb and Donald C. Sheppard, "The Role of Mast Cells in the Defence against Pathogens,"

PLOS Pathogens, 2012 April: 8(4), and Kawa Amin, "The Role of Mast Cells in Allergic Inflammation," *Respiratory Medicine,* January 2012.]

Most people are familiar with the effect mast cells have in the nasal passage where they can cause sneezing and a runny nose. Mast cells are also found in the gut where, when activated, they trigger stomach cramps. For me, mast cells can cause gastrointestinal disorders including hypersensitivity and dysmotility (improper function of the stomach muscles).

Kang Nyeong Lee and Oh Young Lee, writing for *Gastroenterology Research and Practice* in 2016, found that, "Studies have shown an increased number of mast cells in the gut of people who have problems such as IBS." (Lee and Lee, "The Role of Mast Cells in Irritable Bowel Syndrome.") Quercetin has helped tremendously when I have had an inflamed GI tract.

Gastrocrom

Like Quercetin, the prescription medication Gastrostomy (cromolyn sodium) works well for me. The drug is also a mast cell stabilizer but has increased so dramatically in price I only use it in instances when a GI flare-up resists other treatments I try.Gastrocrom specifically treats an overabundance of mast cells called mastocytosis, which causes diarrhea, stomach/abdominal pain, itching, rash, and flushing. (See: "Gastrocrom," *WebMD*, webmd.com.)

Few side effects are reported with Gastrocrom. These include muscle aches, headache, and diarrhea—which could be symptoms of the stomach problem itself. I have experienced none of these issues after taking the medication many times.

UltraMeal and UltraInflamX

UltraMeal and UltraInflamX were formulated to provide macro- and micronutrient support for patients with compromised gut function due to inflammatory bowel disease, ulcerative colitis and Crohn's disease.

The nutrients in these products are broken down to aid in digestion by individuals with gut problems. The combination of the two drinks taken daily stopped the constant IBS attacks I endured for months after my stomach bleed.

Probiotics

I take a comprehensive blend of probiotics daily to maintain high levels of "good" gut bacteria and use a formula that also repopulates the gut. This helps to prevent the overgrowth of yeast, especially while taking an antibiotic, which can kill probiotics. Among its many benefits, acidophilus supports the immune system and improves IBS symptoms. I found high potency probiotics by consulting with my doctor or a licensed nutritionist at a reputable health food store.

Leaky Gut Syndrome

When the lining of the small intestine becomes damaged and porous, a condition called leaky gut syndrome develops. Undigested food particles, toxic waste products and bacteria "leak" through the intestinal walls and flood the bloodstream.

The body tags these particles as foreign invaders and produces antibodies to attack them. When the particles are foods, the body flags them, later causing an allergic reaction when those items are consumed again.

I don't believe the conventional theory that the body is mysteriously attacking itself. Something else is going on. That "something" is what I want to treat. I use my diet and other treatments noted here to heal the gut.

Some strategies that can help include eliminating alcohol, processed foods and addressing any food sensitivities such as the common culprits, gluten and dairy.(See: Matthew Solan, "Putting a Stop to

Leaky Gut," *Harvard Health Publishing: Harvard Medical School*, 18 November 2018.)

Rotation Diet

The rotation diet, which I use when I have frequent flare-ups, helps to prevent reactions to offending foods. I don't eat the same food every day, but instead, I rotate individual items every four days. This period is of sufficient length to allow the food to normally pass through the body's digestive system. Eating the food before it completely leaves the body increases the risk of developing a sensitivity to it. For instance, if I eat apples on Monday, I don't eat them again until Friday.

The Elimination-Challenge Diet

The elimination-challenge diet is a system that can be done at home to help identify offending foods. I prefer to be tested at my doctor's office, either through skin testing or blood tests to find the offending foods. I think it is more accurate. But I have tested foods at home and found the system helpful.

I always check with my doctor first, however, as there can be problems. For example, I was told that it is not safe to do the challenge if I had severe or life-threatening reactions to foods like shrimp or peanuts.

To do the elimination-challenge diet, I removed suspicious foods from my diet for more than four days and then reintroduced the foods one at a time on an empty stomach and watched for adverse reactions. If I have a reaction, I take Alka Seltzer Gold to relieve the symptoms.

However, it was suggested that I should first test the foods I love the most and would least like to give up. These have been found to be the foods most likely to be causing the reactions. That tells me the answer without doing the elimination-challenge diet and is a much easier and safer way to help identify offending foods. Either way, once I identify the offending foods, I can rotate them to prevent future reactions.

GERD/Reflux

Over the years, the minor gastroesophageal reflux disease (GERD) I experienced with upper gastric burning worsened. This occurs when the valve between the esophagus and stomach weakens.

Normally the valve opens to allow food to go down and then shuts tightly. When it does not, stomach acids flow back into the esophagus, causing heartburn or a burning sensation in the upper chest. GERD can also cause chest pain.

Recently I learned I have a hiatal hernia which only makes the symptoms worse. Part of my stomach pushes upward into an opening in the diaphragm, the muscle between the stomach and chest. I can feel the hernia if I press on the center of my chest below the rib cage. The hernia has caused worse gastric attacks that last for days.

For these reasons I have developed a more targeted action plan. In addition to using an antacid and sometimes Gastrocrom, I immediately switch to a bland diet, consisting of rice, oatmeal, scrambled eggs, potatoes and chicken soup, during an episode.

I never take H2 blockers or proton-pump inhibitors, like Zantac. When used long term, these drugs carry serious side effects and have been linked to a heightened risk for cancer.

Several years ago I did take Zantac after a potent antibiotic irritated my stomach and my usual treatments provided no relief. Severe pain from a urinary tract infection led me to risk the antibiotic. As it turned out, the drug was unnecessary because I did not have an infection but rather a nonbacterial condition called interstitial cystitis. Had my condition been diagnosed correctly, I would not have been given an antibiotic, nor would I have taken it. I did not react well to the Zantac either, even in the short term. Instead, I turned to over-the-counter antacids at the maximum allowed dosage and after a few days felt better.

For more information, see: "FDA Updates and Press Announcements on NDMA in Zantac (ranitidine,)" *U.S. Food & Drug Administration*, fda.gov.

Eric Palmer, "Zantac, Generics Ordered Off the Market After FDA Finds They're a Ticking Time Bomb," *Fierce Pharma*, 1 April 2020.

A Word about Interstitial Cystitis

Interstitial cystitis is a chronic bladder inflammation causing pain that feels like an infection. Antibiotics don't help and, in my case, made the situation worse. Most of the things I do for MVPS help to prevent interstitial cystitis flare-ups.

When I actually do have a urinary tract infection, I have used U-Tract, which can be found in health food stores or online. The product works with nature to rid the urinary tract of E. coli. U-Tract is made from D-Mannose, a natural simple sugar that attaches to the E. coli, causing them to stick to each other rather than the walls of the urinary tract. The bacteria can then easily be eliminated from the body during urination.

For more information, see: Chris Kresser, "Treat and Prevent UTIs Without Drugs," *Kresser Institute*, 22 September 2016.

My Treatment For GERD

When I have a gastritis attack, I take an antacid along with Tri-Salts but not at the same time. My doctor told me to separate the two by at least thirty minutes. I also drink a lot of water to help dilute the acid in my GI tract before I take the antacid.

This system works well for me. When I have spasms and pain in my chest from gastritis, I add Bentyl to my protocol. These interventions can quickly calm down the worst flare-ups. I also have an adjustable bed and sleep with my upper body elevated so the acid can't flow up.

Osteopathic manipulation treatments for my IBS help my lower stomach stay more flexible, which also seems to improve upper GI pain. Overall, getting the GI tract moving helps all my symptoms.

Stool Tests

I thought I knew myself from the inside out, until I did a comprehensive stool analysis. These tests have helped me find and resolve gut problems. Sometimes the test comes back without finding any issues.

But if I have bacteria or yeast at any given time, I need to know in order to understand the health of my GI tract and take the appropriate steps to treat it. With everything else going on with my system, I don't need or want any added problems.

Chapter 14
The Often Overlooked and Undertreated Thyroid and Adrenals

Because the symptoms of thyroid disorders can mimic emotional behaviors, they are often misdiagnosed as emotional problems. The thyroid gland, located in the front of the neck below the larynx, controls all metabolic processes in the body.

The gland secretes the hormones thyroxine (T4) and triiodothyronine (T3). The most common thyroid malfunctions are hypothyroidism, which occurs when the gland makes too little of the thyroid hormones, or hyperthyroidism when it makes too much.

Hypothyroidism

Hypothyroidism, or underactivity of the thyroid gland, causes a variety of symptoms such as:

- depression
- fatigue
- weakness
- cold intolerance
- constipation
- weight gain (unintentional)
- joint or muscle pain
- thin and brittle fingernails
- dry, thin and brittle hair
- pale color
- dry and flaky skin
- puffy hands and feet
- decreased taste and smell
- abnormal menstrual periods

Hyperthyroidism

Hyperthyroidism, or over activity of the thyroid gland, may occur naturally or as a result of taking thyroid medication.

In the latter case, the dosage can be adjusted. Symptoms of too much thyroid hormones are:

- fatigue at the end of the day but difficulty sleeping
- trembling of the hands
- hard or irregular heartbeat (palpitations)
- increased blood pressure
- shortness of breath
- chest pain
- muscle weakness
- irritability and tendency to become easily upset
- increased risk of osteoporosis
- weight loss
- diarrhea
- abdominal cramps
- sweating
- heat intolerance
- menstrual irregularities

The Problem with Lab Tests

The typical blood test used by doctors to measure thyroid stimulating hormone (TSH) often fails to show abnormalities in T3 and T4, two other hormones secreted by the thyroid gland. As my doctor explained the situation to me, someone with normal T3, T4, and TSH may still experience classic thyroid symptoms.

"Normal" values are nothing but averages taken from a collection of individuals presumed to be healthy.

Unhealthy people in the control sample will skew the range. (Ryan Andrews, MS, MA, RD, RYT, CSCS, "Blood Tests & Lab Analysis: How It Works and What You Need to Know," *Precision Nutrition*.)

At best, basic laboratory tests are screening devices that provide a snapshot of what is going on in the body at an instant in time.

That is why some good doctors will treat the patient who has symptoms of low thyroid hormones instead of depending only on the lab report.

Before modern lab tests existed, thyroid problems were diagnosed more by physical symptoms after a complete examination. If the patient's symptoms resolved while taking thyroid medication, the diagnosis was made, and the treatment was continued. [Raphael Kellman, MD, Contributor, "Why Routine Blood Tests Often Fail to Detect Low Thyroid Function (And What We Can Do About It)," *Huffington Post*, huffpost.com, 10 May 2015.]

Other Ways to Test Thyroid

Simple temperature readings are also an indicator of thyroid function. My doctor recommended that I take my basal body temperature, the body's morning temperature at the time of awakening but before getting out of bed or moving around.

I shook down a glass thermometer the night before and placed it next to my bed. In the morning, I put the thermometer under my armpit and lay still for ten minutes. I did this for two mornings in a row. A temperature lower than the range of 97.8 - 98.2 could indicate hypothyroidism, while a higher reading could suggest hyperthyroidism. I tested low.

Iodine Skin Patch Test

Another test I've done involves spreading a small, one-inch patch of common over-the-counter iodine on my inner thigh, arm or abdomen and monitoring how quickly my body absorbs it for use.

The iodine is supposed to last twenty-four hours. If it does not, the result suggests low iodine, which is necessary for the thyroid to function. Iodine is added to salt for this very reason.

In theory, since everyone eats salt, everyone gets iodine to make the thyroid gland function. Since many people have been told to cut back on salt to help control blood pressure, however, sodium is not present in the average diet at levels once considered "normal."

Additional dietary sources of iodine may be needed. Kelp is one source and can be taken as a nutritional supplement. Iodine can be prescribed, or SSKI (potassium iodide solution)

(For more information, see: David Brownstein, *Iodine: Why You Need It, Why You Can't Live Without It*, Medical Alternative Press, 1 January 2014.

I Am Unique

I am the best test for whether I need to take thyroid medication or not. I take T3 and T4 daily and have felt much better since I began the treatment. That's the only test that matters to me.

Although there are various thyroid formulations, taking T3 and T4 separately works for me. Some drugs, like Armour Thyroid or Thyrolar, combine both. That helps many people but was not effective for me. According to my doctor, it is not uncommon for people to try a variety of thyroid medications before finding the one that works best.

For more information on the thyroid, see:
Robert M. Sargis MD, PhD, "Thyroid Gland Overview," *Endocrine Web*, endocrineweb.com.

Adrenal Fatigue

The adrenal glands sit on top of the kidneys and produce cortisol when the body is under stress. When these glands become fatigued, people can feel depressed. This should be a short-term reaction, but my MVPS adrenal problems cause my adrenals to overwork almost daily.

To try to counteract fatigue, some people exercise excessively, seeking a "runner's high," or find other ways to increase their cortisol levels. This will also cause exhaustion after the fact.

I was always overreacting, trying to stay excited about anything and everything. This was my typical path to increased cortisol levels, which also helped me feel energized. The effort was exhausting.

The result was a feeling familiar to some MVPS patients—"wired but tired." Any method to increase cortisol will eventually cause further depletion of adrenal function. Treating that depletion with a replacement dose or physiological dose of cortisol has given me energy without pushing my adrenals. Mainstream medicine does not recognize adrenal fatigue.

Take for instance the material provided on the Mayo Clinic website about the condition: "Adrenal fatigue isn't an accepted medical diagnosis. It is a lay term applied to a collection of nonspecific symptoms, such as body aches, fatigue, nervousness, sleep disturbances and digestive problems." (Ann Kearns, M.D., Ph.D., "Adrenal Fatigue: What Causes It?" *Mayo Clinic,* mayoclinic.org.)

A problem I have is discounted with no offer of help for my symptoms. When I did seek help for low energy and fatigue, I am yet again confronted with a diagnosis of depression.

In my opinion, such an unfounded diagnosis discounts the patient and represents another win for the antidepressant industry. Fortunately my doctors do recognize adrenal fatigue and have treated it.

About the Treatment

My adrenal fatigue is treated with a low, "physiological dose" of hydrocortisone—just enough to replace what my body no longer makes.

High therapeutic levels of cortisone are used to treat inflammation and other symptoms on a short-term basis. Used in the long term, such doses carry serious side effects such as:

- osteoporosis
- ulcers
- cataracts
- glaucoma
- menstrual irregularities
- diabetes

Cortisone can suppress growth in children, decrease carbohydrate tolerance, impair wound healing, and suppress the immune system. These effects can continue even after the drug is stopped.

The low replacement dose I take is comparable to insulin replacement for diabetes, hormone replacement therapy (HRT) for menopausal women, and, of course, thyroid replacement. Cortisone has been found to be safe when given in the correct physiological dose to those individuals with malfunctioning adrenal glands.

For more information, see: William Jeffries, *Safe Uses of Cortisone*, Charles C Thomas Pub Ltd; 2nd edition, 1 July 1996. At the time of this publication, this book could be found at used bookstores online.

Chapter 15
My Doctor Found It:
I Have A MTHFR Gene Mutation

In 2013, my doctor ordered a new blood test for the MTHFR genotype. The results showed that I have a mutation in that gene, which, if not addressed, can cause many MVPS problems as well as others that are much more serious.

An estimated 30%-40% of all people may carry an inherited MTHFR gene mutation. The methylenetetrahydrofolate reductase gene (MTHFR) regulates the processing of folate and other B vitamins essential to break down and convert homocysteine into other substances the body needs.

After this process, little homocysteine should remain in the bloodstream. The enzyme, however, has the potential to mutate, which can inhibit the breakdown of homocysteine, causing a buildup in the blood called hyperhomocysteinemia.

Various disorders can then result, affecting the:

- Eyes
- Joints
- Cognitive abilities
- It can cause an increased risk for:
- Heart disease
- Stroke
- High blood pressure
- Blood clots
- Birth defects
- Autoimmune disorders.*

(*An instance in which the immune system attacks healthy tissues. An example would be rheumatoid arthritis.)

Fibromyalgia and myalgic encephalomyelitis/chronic fatigue syndrome are not yet accepted as autoimmune diseases, but there is some discussion about how each shares feature with such disorders.

In the future, there may even be a link drawn between homocysteine levels and these chronic problems.

Given the thin line often drawn between such distinctions, I feel that treating my MTHFR mutation is another way I may be helping the MVPS symptoms, especially as there is no downside to the strategy.

I take supplements of vitamin B and folate to counter the potential issues caused by the mutations, but these must be methylated formulations since I cannot methylate well on my own.

Knowing about the MTHFR gene and treating it correctly is another example of why I am so fortunate to have found progressive physicians who are always researching and learning to find new and better ways to help their patients.

For more information regarding the MTHFR mutation and associated issues, see the following sources:

"MTHFR Mutation Test: What is an MTHFR Mutation Test?" *MedlinePlus,* medlineplus.gov.

Ashley Marcin, "What You Need to Know About the MTHFR Gene," *Healthline,* 6 September 2019.

Jamie Eske, "What is an MTHFR Mutation?" *Medical News Today,* 29 August 2019.

S. Brustolin, R. Giugliani, and T. M. Félix, "Genetics of Homocysteine Metabolism and Associated Disorders," *Brazilian Journal of Medical and Biological Research,* 4 December 2009.

"Myalgic Encephalomyelitis/Chronic Fatigue Syndrome," *Centers for Disease Control and Prevention,* cdc.gov.

Chapter 16
Breakthrough Treatments
That Changed My Life

While searching for answers for my MVPS symptoms, I began to feel as if I were playing a game of Whac-A-Mole. Every attempt to solve one problem turned out to be a temporary improvement, and then a new symptom would pop up. When I fixed that one, the previous symptom would pop up again. I hit the same targets over and over again, gaining some relief, but I never completely won the game.

Without a doubt, the treatments I tried significantly improved the quality of my life. My symptoms occurred less frequently and decreased in duration. Sometimes I could feel them coming on and stop the flare-up before it occurred.

I felt better and more in control but I was determined to end the futile game once and for all. I continued to search for the cause of the sporadic flare-ups, but I was not successful until a new and more formidable health crisis forced the issue.

The Worst Symptoms Ever

The roof over my garage developed a major leak. The flat-top roof, sealed with tar, completely detached from the back wall of the garage. Water poured in during every rain, causing extensive damage.

Mold covered the wet wood, which needed to be replaced. I spent several months searching for a nontoxic roofing material, a necessary step before I could get a restoration company to professionally remove the mold.

I interviewed roofing companies and conferred with environmental specialists. I wanted a nontoxic substance that would adhere to the tar and seal the gap, but I wasn't having any luck.

Conventional roofing materials take months to "off-gas," a process during which volatile organic compounds (VOCs) are released into the air we breathe. I was concerned that my house could become filled with toxic fumes.

At the same time, my air conditioning unit had to be replaced. The new unit more efficiently pulled in outside air. The mold smell, previously confined to the garage, filled my living space.

I called a specialist to seal the air spaces from the garage to the house, but the containment measures didn't work. I needed to fix the leak and remediate the garage before I could clean the air in the house. I felt stuck.

Either I would have to smell mold or toxic roofing chemicals. Either would eventually force me to leave my home. I knew I would have to move out and stay with a friend or rent a safe place.

Meanwhile, I started feeling sick from the mold exposure. I had a weird, weak feeling down the right side of my body similar to a migraine only more pronounced. It didn't let up. I thought I was having a transient ischemic attack (TIA) also known as a ministroke.

A TIA occurs when there is a temporary blockage of blood flow to the brain. The incident doesn't cause permanent damage but often warns of a future stroke.

Three fingers on my left hand drooped and were difficult to lift and use. I had the strength to move them, but only with effort. When I wasn't using my hand, my fingers fell limp.

The worst symptom was the weakness in my throat that made swallowing difficult when I was lying down. The sensation of gagging on saliva forced me to sit up all night. I saw two neurologists who told me nothing was wrong.

They both gave me that "look" I used to get in the ER when I would show up repeatedly with benign chest pains.

I was on my own again and even more scared than before. I started researching my symptoms, and the only diagnosis that came up over and over again was multiple sclerosis (MS).

MS damages the protective coverings of nerve cells, reducing function in the brain and spinal cord, causing:

- Fatigue
- Numbness
- Pain
- Spasms
- Paralysis
- Diminished brain function

A diagnosis can take years. There are no specific tests for MS. The presence of MS is only determined by ruling out other conditions that produce similar symptoms.

(See: "Multiple Sclerosis: Diagnosis," *Mayo Clinic*, mayoclinic.org.)

When I read that mold exposure can trigger MS symptoms, I began to think my problems stemmed from a reaction to the mold, not the onset of a disease.

I needed to stop focusing on the symptoms and fix the problem— mold. First, I had to decide on a roof, even one constructed of toxic materials, to stop the leaks. Then, and only then, the mold could be removed. Once back home, I stood a better chance of resting and healing.

Choosing the least toxic material I could find, I was encouraged to learn the roof would off-gas faster during the hot Texas summer with the fumes likely being drawn into the atmosphere, not the garage. It worked.

The roofing materials did not smell inside, and the leaks were sealed. Hired professionals removed the mold from the garage, and the musty smell in the house which had been caused by spores being pulled through the air conditioning.

Everything had to be washed down. We washed all the walls, floors, clothing, linens, even the pencils on my desk. The process was overwhelming, but with the help of a friend, we got it done.

A machine that generates ozone eradicated the remaining mold odor left in the air, crevices, and furniture. The devices, used in hospitals, hotels, and homes, kill not only mold spores and cells but also bacteria and odors such as smoke.

I could not be in the house during the treatment. Ozone removes all oxygen during the process. When completed, I had the air tested again, which showed the mold levels were back to normal. I returned home, but a faint smell of mold lingered. According to the Environmental Protection Agency (EPA), a moldy odor suggests that mold is still growing.

(See: "What Does Mold Smell Like?" *United States Environmental Protection Agency*, epa.gov.)

I hoped the smell would die off or that it would not affect me. I was wrong. The odor remained and so did my symptoms. Then I got worse.

While I was driving home from an errand, my left hand suddenly froze. I could not bend my fingers, nor could I grip the steering wheel. I panicked. My right side was still weak, including the leg I used to press the brake.

I pulled over, holding my claw-like, rigid hand up in front of my face, trying to make the fingers move. They wouldn't. I called a friend to let him know where I was and told him I would try to drive home on back roads. He met me at my house and took me to the ER. By the time we got there, the movement in my hand had almost completely returned but some stiffness remained. The ER doctor was kind. After running some tests and observing me for a couple of hours, he decided the incident represented a variation of my migraine headaches.

I left the hospital, but I knew what happened was part of a slew of new symptoms that occurred after my exposure to mold. Clearly, the problem was not going away on its own. If anything, it was getting worse. I had to find a way to stop it.

That was when I discovered a breakthrough program that addressed the cause of all my chronic symptoms from the mold exposure *and* those caused by MVPS. Now, armed with this program and two others, I have the tools to improve my health and life at any time.

Treatment 1:
Dynamic Neural Retraining System™

I turned to one of my good doctors for help with my mold problem. He told me about a new program developed by Annie Hopper called the Dynamic Neural Retraining System™ (DNRS).

He heard Hopper speak at an American Academy of Environmental Medicine (AAEM) conference where she described a nondrug approach to facilitate recovery from intractable medical problems such as chemical, electrical and food sensitivities, chronic fatigue syndrome, fibromyalgia and more.

Hopper's work is based on neuroplasticity, the theory that the brain can "rewire" itself in response to a variety of factors, including chronic illness and trauma. Her program retrains the brain to correct chronic disease patterns. Basically, if the brain can learn to be ill, it can learn to be well.

Rewiring the Brain

As an example of brain rewiring, consider how actor Leonardo DiCaprio prepared for his award-nominated role as Howard Hughes in *The Aviator*. In his later years, Hughes suffered with obsessive-compulsive disorder (OCD), a condition that causes fears and unrelenting, repetitive behaviors.

DiCaprio learned how OCD felt and how to behave as if he had the disorder. He taught himself to be a person with OCD. The result was a stunning and accurate portrayal that left DiCaprio with a mild version of the disorder that required months of recovery.

The actor's conscious plunge into OCD and later recovery illustrates neuroplasticity—the ability of the brain to change. Dr. Jeffrey Schwartz, the therapist and author of *Brain Lock*, helped DiCaprio learn and unlearn OCD.

(For an account of DiCaprio's experience see: Steve Volk, "Rewiring the Brain to Treat OCD," *Discover*, 10 December 2013.)

The Limbic System

Annie Hopper's program targets the limbic system, the part of the brain that assigns emotional significance to everything we smell, see, hear, feel, and taste. The limbic system forms memories and determines our level of safety.

The limbic system can become impaired by:

- Chemical exposure
- Mold toxicity
- A virus or infection
- Inflammation

- Psychological and/or emotional trauma
- Accumulated stress
- Physical trauma

When this occurs, the person becomes unconsciously stuck in a state of fight or flight—what Hopper calls a "trauma loop." A wide variety of negative symptoms then become chronic.

At the time of this publication, Hopper's presentation at the AAEM conference, "Limbic Rehabilitation: A Novel Treatment Approach for Lifestyle Exposure Related Neurotoxicity," was available on the Dynamic Neural Retraining System YouTube channel.

After viewing the presentation, I came to believe a limbic system dysfunction was affecting me.

Even though the mold exposure was gone, my body was responding as if it was still there.

That might have been why I could smell mold even though the air quality testing following the remediation showed normal levels. My sensitivity to mold had become so severe I reacted to the low levels common in most homes. Protective mechanisms in my brain responded to the hypersensitivity by overfiring, resulting in distorted, unconscious reactions and responses.

I signed up for the next workshop which was two months away in Santa Fe. Even though I felt bad and was dealing with scary symptoms, I was determined to travel anywhere for her program, which I saw as possibly my only hope and certainly my best chance to recover.

Physically, the trip was the hardest I've ever made, but emotionally, it was the easiest. I was tired, weak and never sure I could control my body. If I was going to die, I decided I could do it in Santa Fe or on the plane trying to get there rather than sit passively waiting in a state of panic in my toxic house.

I arrived in Santa Fe weak and unsteady, wondering if I had the stamina to get through the program or even get home on my own if the process didn't work fast enough.

Sitting in the lobby, meeting and visiting with other participants who had also just arrived, I looked at my left hand resting on the arm of the chair and hoped it would move at my command. I remember my relief when it did. My symptoms were full-blown. My body didn't feel real or even connected to me—and I was overcome with fear.

By the time I left five days later, I was almost back to my old self. I continued to do the program at home to develop and strengthen the new healthier brain pathways I had developed, but I was well on my way.

Today, the MS symptoms are gone. After more than six years, they've never returned. I also targeted my MVPS symptoms with the same system and enjoyed excellent results. Annie Hopper's website says, "Retrain Your Brain, Transform Your Health and Reclaim Your Life." I can say unequivocally, from my personal experience, her program worked for me.

For more information on the DNRS program,
see: RetrainingTheBrain.com.

Treatment 2:
SOAR and Panic Free Program

Flying never worried me until after the 9/11 attack. Timing is everything when it comes to the limbic system. My brother, who lived alone in Florida, had a heart attack, and I needed to fly there to help him.

It was only two weeks after 9/11, and I was not ready to get on an airplane again. The flight was almost empty—literally. There were fewer than ten passengers.

The large Dallas/Fort Worth International Airport was almost deserted. Clearly, I was not alone in my concerns and felt an intense uneasiness on that flight that would later usher in a full-blown phobia.

The plane took off, and I felt the first pangs of panic. Looking back, I can see that my uneasiness and the raw terror of 9/11 fired together and were, from that moment forward, wired together.

I became a very nervous flyer. It did not help that all my life I had watched my mother avoid flying out of fear, something she often told me. Consequently, the first twinges of apprehension appeared even before 9/11. I was primed to become the proverbial nervous flyer.

After that trip, I avoided flying whenever I could. If I had to get on a plane, I experienced mild anxiety the entire time mixed with moments of panic caused by any noise or bumpy movements. I remained in that state from the time the plane took off until the wheels hit the ground and the brakes slowed the forward motion.

I tried a variety of hypnosis tapes. They didn't work. I consulted a talented hypnotherapist who had successfully helped me stop my arrhythmias, but he couldn't help me either.

Next, I tried a weekend course for nervous flyers offered by American Airlines. The class ended with a one-hour round-trip graduation flight. I snapped the rubber band on my wrist, bounced in my seat to override the turbulence, tapped my foot on the solid floor, and tried to talk to others in the class as a distraction. Over and over I reminded myself that flying is the safest mode of transportation. Nothing I learned from the class helped—not that day or later.

I lived this way for years and continued to search for help. I happened to find a course called SOAR, taught by retired captain and therapist, Tom Bunn, a man I found to be kind, calming and dynamic.

I talked to him before purchasing the home program and at other times when I had questions. He was always available.

His guarantee sealed the deal for me. *"If you are not satisfied with the improvement when you fly, you will receive a full refund."* No fear-of-flying program I had investigated ever offered a refund.

Fearful flyers are notoriously difficult to cure. If Captain Tom was that certain his program would help, I figured his approach had to be different—boy was I right.

His materials not only explained the source of my fear, but how it targeted the emotional side of my brain. The program teaches that if we become too revved up, we may become unable to differentiate between reality and the stories we make up in our heads. It was as if Captain Tom knew me.

In addition to being a journalist, I am also a playwright. I make up stories all the time and bring them to life on stage. In real life, I can make up the worst-case scenarios for any situation and scare myself to death. Before traveling, I would visualize in great detail how the plane would go down and how it would feel. This story bathed my brain in more and more of the wrong kind of chemicals until my conscious mind couldn't override their effects.

Captain Tom explains the chain of events in this way. When we think "what if" something bad could happen, we trigger the release of stress hormones. The more we think, the more hormones are released and build up in our systems, making us feel tense. Heart rate goes up. Breathing changes. Sweating often occurs. The body recognizes these feelings as indications of danger. In this instance, feeling is believing. We think what we fear might happen *will* happen.

Books and Programs by Captain Tom Bunn

The Program: SOAR: Fear of Flying Course

The Book: SOAR: The Breakthrough Treatment for Fear of Flying

Panic Free: The 10-Day Program to End Panic, Anxiety, and Claustrophobia

Helpful Articles by Captain Tom Bunn:

"Temperament and Anxiety," SOAR Fear of Flying Blog at capt-tom.blogspot.com.

"Fear Can Make You Believe the Worst Will Happen. How?" *Psychology Today*, 16 December 2015.

"A Primer on Psychological Defenses. We all use defenses to alter reality. The question is how severely." *Psychology Today*. August 27, 2021.

The SOAR training helps to prevent panic and fear from building up. Once I am in a full-blown panic attack, it's very hard for me to calm myself. Captain Tom teaches systems that work almost automatically to prevent my fear from ever reaching that point.

The program addressed the emotional side of the fear and also spoke to the logical side of my brain. The course taught me everything about how the plane works. Years after completing the work, I was flying with a friend who had traveled all over the world. After she heard a weird noise, she thought out loud, "What was that?" Not only could I tell her what it was but also that it was normal because I learned all about it in the SOAR course. I didn't really notice the noise that got her attention. I used to be a person who listened for every sound a plane can make during every flight.

I always thought that Captain Tom's program had broader applications for anxiety and panic in general. I have used some of his tools to help reduce my other fears and the adrenaline they provoked.

His recent book, *Panic Free: The 10-Day Program to End Panic, Anxiety, and Claustrophobia*, served as a guide to apply what I learned about my fear of flying to other apprehensions in my everyday life, especially those that relate to my MVPS symptoms.

How the SOAR Fear of Flying Course Works

Where the DNRS program focuses on rewiring the brain, the SOAR course more directly reconnects scary thoughts to safer and happier ones. Both affect the wiring in the brain but via different methods.

SOAR is fast. DNRS can take a few months to take full effect although I did start to feel better immediately. In my experience, the two programs strengthen one another.

"Panic Free with Tom Bunn: How To Stop Panic Attacks," Corinne Zupko YouTube Channel.

Treatment 3:
Mind Over Medicine

In the book, *Mind Over Medicine*, Dr. Lissa Rankin makes a strong argument for taking care of ourselves both physically and emotionally, two approaches I believe were critical in helping me to heal.

As a young woman, Rankin ignored small symptoms until they grew into more serious chronic conditions like high blood pressure, cardiac arrhythmias and debilitating allergies.

During the process of restoring her health, Rankin realized that the conventional medicine she had been taught to practice did not recognize the body's innate ability to repair itself or the healing power we each possess within ourselves.

My MVPS action plan includes the same three-pronged approach she explains. Reading her excellent book reaffirmed my decision to live a healthy lifestyle, to choose medical interventions carefully and to develop my innate ability to heal using the breakthrough treatments I've described here.

Groundbreaking Programs

I believe we are on a new frontier of understanding how the brain works and the effect it can have on our health both good and bad. The placebo effect is one example of the power of the mind that has been used for decades.

A placebo is a substance or treatment that has no therapeutic value, but when a patient is told the "drug" can help, it does. The theory holds that the patient's expectation of benefit makes the placebo effective. That is the power of the mind. (Kendra Cherry, "What is the Placebo Effect?" *VeryWellMind.com*, 12 February 2021.)

Today I have found even better tools to accomplish good health. I have learned how to make these kinds of changes in my brain. I am an example that we all have the ability to retrain or rewire the brain.

The change didn't come naturally to me, but I was able, with the aid of excellent teachers, to learn the invaluable process that helped to stop my symptoms and fears.

I believe we stand poised at the brink of a new age of using the brain's plasticity to address thoughts and habits that make people like me sick. This approach may well be the ultimate treatment for MVPS—it's already helping for me.

Chapter 17

MVPS and Postural Tachycardia Syndrome (POTS)

As far back as I can remember I would see spots in front of my eyes whenever I stood up quickly. First I would see the spots in my peripheral vision, but as the number of spots increased, they moved across my eyes until they obstructed my entire vision. Then the spots would rapidly dissipate almost immediately. It felt like a screen wipe in a movie where one scene wipes across the screen to another scene by fading in and out, and I was in that dark place in between for only a second or two. I never felt weak or scared. In fact, I thought it was normal and never complained about it. I rarely experience the spots anymore, but I do sometimes feel a little dizzy when standing up quickly, so the issue still exists.

But for some people it can be a daily problem that does not easily resolve after standing. People with this condition are often diagnosed with postural tachycardia syndrome or POTS, which is considered an autonomic problem affecting the regulation of blood flow. For these people, the longer they are upright, the more blood pools toward the lower part of their body, causing a variety of difficult symptoms with the most common being a rapid heartbeat or tachycardia. This can occur not only when standing up but also when just changing positions while lying down.

Adrenaline

When blood pools in the lower part of the body and does not return to the brain, the body's safety mechanisms will jump in to help by releasing adrenaline. The adrenaline tightens the blood vessels to help them do their job and send blood back to the brain. But as I have discussed in this book, adrenaline also causes shakiness, pounding or skipped heartbeats, chest pain and may trigger more MVPS symptoms as is typical for me.

POTS and My MVPS Action Plan

So realizing that I am somewhat affected by POTS, the treatments and recommendations for it were of interest to me while developing my action plan.

As I researched POTS, I realized that most of my treatments for MVPS/D were either recommended for POTS or helpful for it. That makes sense to me in that POTS is often associated with MVPS. In my research, I learned that people diagnosed with POTS also report other forms of dysautonomia, and dealing with dysautonomia has been the focus of my action plan.

In addition, the overlap with MVPS symptoms is obvious when looking at the symptoms of POTS.

- Symptoms of POTS include:
- Palpitations
- Light-headedness
- Difficulty breathing
- Chest pain
- Headaches/migraines
- Shakiness
- Sleep problems
- Mental fog
- Exercise intolerance
- Chronic fatigue
- GI Problems

Lifestyle recommendations are also similar to those for MVPS. People with POTS are advised to avoid alcohol, sugar, caffeine and extreme heat, but to include drinking more water, doing mild exercise, eating a balanced diet high in fiber and increasing sodium.

Conventional Treatments for POTS

Although I have included information on a breakthrough treatment for POTS later in this chapter, I usually start my research by learning what is available in conventional medicine. The common and more conventional treatment for POTS is medication. This includes salt tablets to help retain fluid, fludrocortisone to help decrease the amount of sodium that is excreted in the urine, pyridostigmine to help decrease muscle weakness, midodrine, used to treat low blood pressure and/or a beta blocker. In addition, compression stockings are used to help push the blood up from the legs. There is a considerable list of drugs that can make POTS worse. See more information on drugs to avoid at the American Heart Association Journal website.

Mast Cells and POTS

During a joint meeting with patients at a Mastocytosis Society conference, physicians noted a potential connection between mast cell issues and people diagnosed with POTS. Mast cells are part of the immune system that, when activated, release histamine in response to an antigen or a foreign substance. It is similar to experiencing sneezing and a runny nose during an allergic reaction. Most people are familiar with the effect mast cells have in the nasal passages, but mast cells are also found in other parts of the body, including the gut, lungs, skin and around blood vessels. An overactivation of mast cells in any of these areas can cause inflammation resulting in a variety of symptoms. (See: "Gastrocrom," *WebMD*, webmd.com.)

Treatment

I take the prescription, Gastrocrom (cromolyn sodium) to control my IBS symptoms. Cromolyn sodium helps to stabilize mast cells in the gut to relieve stomach problems like diarrhea, pain, nausea, and vomiting. It also helps relieve flushing, headaches, and itching. Quercetin, sold over-the-counter as a dietary supplement, is also a mast cell stabilizer. If I am experiencing any mast cell issues like people diagnosed with POTS, then at least I know that I am helping to relieve the effects since I already take cromolyn sodium daily for my MVPS/D symptoms. See more on Cromolyn Sodium and Quercetin in Chapter 13: Why I Feel It in My Gut and How I Treat IBS, GERD and Gastritis.

The Adrenaline Connection

Another benefit to controlling mast cells is to prevent the release of adrenaline. Here's how it works. During an allergic reaction, the body releases histamine. It then tries to reduce the histamine by releasing adrenaline. Avoiding allergens or treating them as soon as possible can help prevent the flooding of adrenaline into the system. I discuss more on this in Chapter 11: Taking the Fear Out of Anxiety.

A Breakthrough Treatment

I met one person with POTS when I attended The Dynamic Neural Retraining System (DNRS) program that is explained in Chapter 16: Breakthrough Treatments That Changed My Life. Before she did the DNRS home program, she was confined to a reclining wheelchair, unable to even sit upright. Once the home program helped her become mobile, she signed up to take the "in-person" course that I attended and where we met. She was doing so well that she was able to fly to another city to attend the course. She continued to get better during the five-day conference.

The program, however, takes diligence to continue the training practices at home for several months to a year to optimize the benefits. There are several videos and testimonials on the DNRS website of other people with POTS who took the program. There is a video of another young woman with POTS who had also been confined to a reclining wheelchair before the program. Her story and recovery can be viewed at:

https://www.youtube.com/watch?v=jBM7C9UnB8s&t=1s.

The DNRS program, which helped me recover from some devastating symptoms, is designed to retrain the brain from a state of illness to that of health. The website explains the program as follows:

We directly target brain function and a maladapted stress response that is at the root of suffering for so many. We do not chase your symptoms – we teach you how to change the function and structure of your brain. When you rewire the limbic system, you move your body from a state of survival to a state of growth and repair – where true healing can take place.

https://retrainingthebrain.com

Chapter 18
The Basics: My Action Plan for Staying Healthy

Regardless of the time and effort I put into finding new and better options for my MVPS symptoms, I still forget to take care of myself in general. It's easy to skip exercise or to eat unhealthy comfort food when I don't feel well. Even though I can fall off the wagon, I follow a basic, foundational plan that grounds me and supports all my other treatments.

Diet

As the basis of my healthy diet, I don't eat processed foods, fast foods, gluten or beef. I choose organic items almost 100% of the time while avoiding sugar, coffee, and alcohol. I will use small amounts of sweetened chocolate to relieve migraine auras and sometimes opt for small amounts of natural sweeteners like organic honey.

Nutrients

In consultation with my doctor, I take magnesium, folate, and vitamin D. I would like to take vitamin C but can only tolerate it when my GERD is well under control. Instead, I get vitamin C and vitamin B complex with my magnesium IVs.

In addition, I want to try CoQ10 again for the many heart-related benefits, but the first two brands I tried caused headaches. I hope to find a formulation that does not.

Exercise

I pace myself when exercising. If I push too hard with running or walking, I can take as long as a day to recover. For most of my adult life I've been very active and have been able to get in excellent shape without endurance exercises.

Whenever I read articles on exercising safely with MVP, I check with my doctor to determine the best options. I completely avoid any weightlifting, which puts stress on the heart. In my case, weightlifting seemed to trigger autonomic nervous system instability, leaving me light-headed, weak, and often with a headache.

I enjoy yoga, which has gently helped to increase my strength. I also like to walk, and when I can't, I use floor exercises from videos to help me get cardio without overexerting.

A comfortable level of exercise can make me feel good and energetic. I stop before I push too far. I have learned that I can increase my exercise if I progress slowly.

For more information on exercise, see: "5 Exercises to Avoid with Mitral Valve Prolapse," *MVP Resource*, mvpresource.com, 15 October 2017.

Relaxation

Meditation and hypnosis work well for me to reduce or alleviate stress. As I've gotten older, I don't sleep as well or as long, but I have adapted. Since I work at home, I can sleep longer in the morning and get enough hours to feel good and productive. I am always looking for better systems to improve my sleep.

Stress

If I have a concern about a new symptom or an MVPS flare-up, I deal with it rather than worry. I used to wait out such episodes hoping they would go away, putting myself under unnecessary stress.

Knowing the nature of the problem and how to address it creates far less stress than sitting and worrying. I review my notes or research the problem and, when needed, make an appointment with my doctor. If I can't see him or her, I ask for a phone conference.

Worry triggers adrenaline, which always makes my symptoms worse. Nonproductive worry isn't good for me emotionally, but action and a plan always help me more effectively get through health problems.

Avoid Being Overweight

As I have gotten older, an underactive thyroid has made controlling my weight more challenging. Still, too many extra pounds make everything feel worse, especially my GERD and hiatal hernia. I don't need to be as thin as I was most of my life, but currently just being reasonably trim and fit works well for my health.

A Word about Fragrances

Sensitivity to artificial chemicals can trigger my MVPS symptoms, but many of these substances aren't good for anyone. Ninety-five percent of synthetic fragrances are made from petroleum chemicals (crude oil) that have a negative effect on the nervous system. Irritation of the throat and stomach can also occur as well as difficulty breathing. ("Ingredient Watch List: Synthetic Fragrance Exposes You to Hundreds of Chemicals," *AnnMarieGianni.com*, 1 May 2018.)

"The Environmental Working Group blames the U.S. government in part, pointing out that the Food and Drug Administration 'has not assessed the safety of the vast majority of secret chemicals used in spray-on products such as fragrances.'" Unless the label says natural or organic fragrances, the product probably contains synthetic fragrances.

Although not always listed, these fragrances are usually made from petrochemicals. These synthetic fragrances are commonly used in shampoos, hand and body lotions, soaps, hair spray, aftershave sprays and lotions, laundry detergents and deodorants. In addition, they are present in spray and plug-in air fresheners as well as scented candles.

("Scent of Danger: Are There Toxic Ingredients in Perfumes and Colognes?" Scientific American, 29 September 2012.)

Even natural oils used in diffusers can cause illnesses and affect the respiratory system.

Studies show that volatile organic compounds (VOCs) can be released from diffused essential oils, causing increased bronchial hyperresponsiveness among patients with and without asthma. ("Essential Oil Diffusers and Asthma," *American Academy of Allergy, Asthma & Immunology*, aaaai.org, 24 February 2020.)

For more information, see: "Petrochemical Fuel," *Science Direct*, ScienceDirect.com.

Stacy Malkan, "Petroleum in Perfume," *Huffington Post*, 25 May 2011.

"FAQs: Fragrances," *Eco-Healthy Child Care*, cehn.org.

Insecticides

If insecticides are perfectly safe, as we have been assured, then why did the government ban similar poisons in the past, despite previous assurances of their safety?

DDT was used extensively until the chemical was found to have a negative impact on the environment and was linked to tumors in animals. I wonder which insecticides or other chemicals currently being called "safe" will be pulled off the shelves tomorrow? Some substances banned in other countries are still being sold in the United States. (Nathan Donley, "The USA Lags Behind Other

Agricultural Nations in Banning Harmful Pesticides," *Environmental Health,* 7 June 2019.)

Many pesticides still widely used in the United States in great quantities have been banned or are being phased out in the European Union, China and Brazil. Of the pesticides banned in at least two of these places, many have been implicated in acute pesticide poisonings in the U.S., and some are further restricted by individual states. (Nathan Donley, "The USA Lags Behind Other Agricultural Nations in Banning Harmful Pesticides," *Environmental Health,* 7 June 2019.)

Carolyn Gorman, in her 2013 book *Less Toxic Living,* offers a variety of easy recipes for safe bug killers. I make boric acid balls that are incredibly effective in killing roaches and other insects.

She also offers ideas and resources for safer products as options to replace many of the toxic commercial products used today. Gorman is extremely knowledgeable and spent much of her career at the Environmental Health Center in Dallas, Texas. In her capacity as a consultant, she helped me research roofing material during my mold problem.

The weed killer Roundup, a well-known yard chemical, is still used in the U.S. despite its questionable history. In 2018, Monsanto, the manufacturer of Roundup, lost a $289 million court judgment in favor of cancer patients in multiple states. The court found that Monsanto "acted with malice, oppression or fraud and should be punished for its conduct." (Michael James and Jorge L. Ortiz, "Jury Orders Monsanto to Pay $289 Million to Cancer Patient in Roundup Lawsuit," *USA Today,* 10 August 2018.)

In my opinion, the chemical marketplace operates on the basis of "buyer beware." The negative effects of these products may only be revealed after they've been used in our homes and environment for years.

I work too hard to stay healthy to undermine my efforts and health by using or being exposed to synthetic chemicals. For general health purposes, there appear to be more reasons than just my MVPS to avoid these substances.

Staying healthy is the most basic piece of my overall action plan to recover from MVPS.

Chapter 19
Taking Control of MVPS:
The Four Best Choices I Ever Made

Everything in this book was designed to help me with my health issues. To develop my action plan, I evaluated all the information I found and judged all my experiences through the lens of my values and opinions.

We are all different even if we may all have MVPS. I am in no way telling anyone how they should feel or what they should do medically to treat their symptoms.

I am not a doctor or an expert on MVPS, but I was able to take steps to care for myself and to become an active participant in my healthcare. This is a choice any patient can make

The Right to Choose

When I talk about my rights as a patient to make decisions, I am not referring to the Patient's Bill of Rights that was adopted by the American Hospital Association. Those rights are actually just a list of promises made by the hospital for the people receiving medical care at that facility. That list also includes rights guaranteed by law that we already possess.

I live in a country where I have the right as an adult to make medical decisions for myself. I do not have to ask for permission from the medical community. I have had to make many important medical decisions on my own.

However, the following four decisions were the most significant. They put me back in control and sent me down a path to finding better treatments for my MVPS symptoms.

1. I Chose Action Over Worry

MVPS symptoms cause a lot of worry. They're scary, unnerving, and sometimes make me feel like I'm dying. Then, capriciously, the symptoms fade, leaving me battered and apprehensive about the next time—and there was always a next time.

I used to refer to the times between MVPS attacks as periods of remission because I knew the respite was only temporary. I was caught in a vicious cycle, worrying about when the symptoms would occur and then about how long it would take for them to end. The worry provoked adrenaline, adding fuel to the fire. Taking action changed that.

First, I learned everything I could about MVPS. Then, I found more helpful doctors. Every appointment I made was actually a job interview. If the physician could help, they were hired. If they had nothing to offer, I moved on.

Taking control gave me a new focus that immediately took my mind off worrying while yielding answers and options that benefited me in the long run.

Looking back, I realize that no one could help me until I decided to help myself.

Even though I have experience researching medical issues, I'm still a patient, not a medical professional. In my opinion, if I can research and find answers, anyone can.

2. I Chose to Learn Everything I Could About MVPS and My Health

The references, links, and details provided in this book are intended to validate the accuracy of the information on which I have based my opinions and treatments. I wanted to demonstrate the importance I placed on this work, but also to document the data for myself. I now have a single place where I can find all my resources should I need them in the future.

Today, with the internet at our fingertips, anyone can do this kind of research. For anyone looking for more answers, many can be found by simply working with a search engine. There are many professionals to consult, including doctors and pharmacists.

The following books have given me a solid overview of MVPS. I refer to them to this day. My copies are highlighted and dog-eared. Both reside on my bedside table.

Hoffman, Ronald. *Natural Therapies for Mitral Valve Prolapse: A Good Health Guide. Keats Good Health Guides.* New York: McGraw Hill, 1 February 1999.

Durante, Cheryl and James F. *The Mitral Valve Prolapse Syndrome/ Dysautonomia Survival Guide.* Oakland: New Harbinger Publications, 11 January 1999.

Another important book specifically addresses anxiety:

Bunn, Tom. *Panic Free: The 10-Day Program to End Panic, Anxiety, and Claustrophobia.* Novato, California: New World Library, 30 April 2019.

When adrenaline pours into my system leaving me feeling shaken and anxious, Bunn's system has been incredibly effective for me. I get his weekly newsletter with current information on calming anxiety and panic. Over the past ten years, I've probably gathered fifteen to twenty books worth of information through those emails.

Anderson, Joan. *My Action Plan for Stopping the Symptoms of MVPS.*
I now add my book to the others. It represents my personal MVPS action plan to remind me of the best steps I can take and the most

effective treatments I can use when needed. In the midst of an MVPS crisis, having this information in one place is invaluable. Before I ever considered writing a book, I kept a spiral notebook and printouts from the internet on my night table that contained all the useful information I had found during my research. It was the beginning of my action plan. All those notes and information became the genesis of this book.

Keeping such a notebook is something I would recommend to anyone working to develop their own MVPS action plan.

3. I Chose to Develop and Use My 5 Patient Principles

Good health is important to me. I work hard to stay healthy. I depend on my 5 Patient Principles to help me get the best medicine has to offer while avoiding the worst. Over the years, my principles have helped me make sound decisions about medical care even when I was scared and not thinking clearly. They may not work for anyone else, nor were they designed to do that. They were developed for me and are based on my core values, my health and medical issues, and my experiences with the medical system.

Principle 1:
MVPS Symptoms Are Physical, Not Emotional
A quick fix with a psychiatric drug does not address the physical problem.

Principle 2:
A Symptom Is a Clue Not a Disease
Find the cause, fix the problem, instead of covering symptoms with drugs.

Principle 3:
Be Sure Tests and Treatments are Necessary and Not Worse Than the Problem

Whether it is a treatment or a test, I want to weigh the risks and benefits. People have died from prescription drugs, surgeries and tests.

Principle 4:
One Protocol Does Not Work for Everyone
Be sure that "standard of care" or "standing orders" or any patient treatment guidelines fit my unique needs. I don't want to be a square peg forced into a round hole. It always makes things worse for me.

Principle 5
Trust Myself
I am an expert too. I know my medical history, my symptoms, how my body works, acts and reacts better than anyone else.

4. I Chose to Take Back My Power and My Legal Rights

I realized early on in my career as a medical reporter that the patient holds the power and control in their hands. For many years I let doctors either make decisions for me or hoped that they would agree with my suggestions. That lasted for thirty years.

I took back my power after a harrowing experience at the hands of a careless, unfeeling doctor during the delivery of my second child. I emerged with my eyes open to the failures of the medical system and fully cognizant that I am responsible for the decisions and consequences of my medical care.

When I am informed and educated about issues that affect me, I can make the best decisions. If I am unable to make choices for myself, I have legally designated a person I trust to do so in my stead through my medical power of attorney (MPOA).

The MPOA documents, which are specific for each state, can be downloaded online at no cost.

Two neighbors witnessed my signature, but the document could also be notarized.

The power of choice belongs to me and the person I designated to act for me, not the doctors, nurses, or hospital.

As a patient of legal age and competence, I have the power to:

- Decide when to access medical care.
- Decide which doctors to hire and pay.
- Leave a hospital or walk out of a doctor's office at any time.
- Research and learn more about my own health issues.
- Choose a healthy lifestyle and diet.
- Take care of my health or not.
- Choose or decline any and all medical care and treatment offered.

This is my body. I own it. I am responsible for it. I found that learning, researching and doing the work to care for myself has been more than worth the effort. With the help of many professionals, the support of my friends and the sharing of information from other MVPS patients, I have slowly worked my way out of the grips of MVPS and taken back my life.

This book is not intended to be a "how-to" manual, but rather an account of the actions I have taken and how they have been of benefit to me. Anyone can do what I did in a way that is specific to their unique situation.

Perhaps this book will inspire you to find your way out of the MVPS maze using a plan based on your personal health issue, values, principles, research and professional input. I wish you good health and relief from your MVPS symptoms.

My Resources

This is a list of some of the tools and resources that I use as explained in the book. Please note that I do not have an affiliate relationship with any of the listed products or authors and receive no compensation for listing these resources. The recommendations reflect my personal experience and use only.

Google Alerts for New Information on MVPS

I signed up on Google Alerts to receive notices of new information on mitral valve prolapse syndrome. Google monitors the web for new content and sends an email to registrants with links to articles.

To create an alert:

1. Go to www.google.com/alerts.
2. In the box, enter a topic you wish to follow.
3. To change settings click "Show Options." You can change:
4. Frequency of notifications.
5. Types of sites you'll see.
6. Language.
7. World regions from which you will receive information.
8. Number of desired results.
9. What Google accounts will receive the alert.
10. Click "Create Alert."

Drug Information Sites

For information on FDA approved drugs, including an overview, side effects, dosage and interactions, see:

Physician Desk Reference – www.pdr.net

Drugs.com – www.drugs.com

RxList - www.rxlist.com

Drug Interactions Checker
https://www.drugs.com/drug_interactions.html
The Drugs.com interaction section allows users to list drugs, which will then be checked for potential negative interactions or other problems caused by taking the medications in combination

Helpful Programs

Dynamic Neural Retraining System – by Annie Hopper

SOAR Fear of Flying Course by Captain Tom Bunn

Helpful Books and Articles

Bunn, Tom. *Panic Free: The 10-Day Program to End Panic, Anxiety, and Claustrophobia.* Novato, California: New World Library, 30 April 2019.

Hoffman, Ronald. *Natural Therapies for Mitral Valve Prolapse: A Good Health Guide. Keats Good Health Guides.* New York: McGraw Hill, 1 February 1999.

Hoffman, Ronald, "Mitral Valve Prolapse," DrHoffman.com, 4 October 2013.

Durante, Cheryl and James F. *The Mitral Valve Prolapse Syndrome/Dysautonomia Survival Guide.* Oakland: New Harbinger Publications, 11 January 1999.)

Products and Labs
For IBS:

UltraInFlamx and UltraMeal
Metagenics Medical Foods

Homeopathic Nausea Drops for Migraine Aura Headaches

Special Order from:
Homeocare Laboratories
7 Odell Plaza, Suite 142
Yonkers NY 10701
www.homeocare.com
(914)-920-5991

Homeopathic Ingredients:
Aethusa cynapium (Fools Parsley) 4x
Podophyllum peltatum (May Apple) 4x
Anacardium orientale (making Nut) 6x
Colchicum autumnale (meadow Saffron) 6x
Ipecacuanha (Ipecac) 6x
Iodium (Iodine) 12x
Other ingredients Purified water and 20% USP alcohol

Tools and Equipment
Fingertip Oximeter which Measures Oxygen Level & Pulse Rate

Omron Home Manual Blood Pressure Kit, Gray

Omron 10 Series Wireless Upper Arm Blood Pressure Monitor

EMAY Portable ECG Monitor

ReadMyHeart Handheld ECG-EKG Monitor F

Salonpas pain relief patch for the temporary relief of mild to moderate muscle and joint aches and pains associated with arthritis, sprains, strains, bruises and simple backache.
I sometimes use these for costochondritis (rib pain).

Bed Buddy®
Microwave Heating Pad for Aches and Pain and Headaches

About the Author
From Medical Journalist to MVPS Patient

Joan Anderson began experiencing symptoms of mitral valve prolapse syndrome before the medical community seemed to know or acknowledge the condition existed. Her doctors just patted her on the head, told her that her palpitations were perfectly normal for an overstressed mother of two and sent her on her way.

Although there was no internet to answer her growing questions, Joan was a journalist and medical writer who was experienced in researching health issues and cutting through barriers to find answers. Joan's approach as a medical reporter was to learn as much as possible about a health problem and then inform the public about its impact on their lives and what they can do to combat it. She took on her personal assignment about MVPS with the same vigor.

Joan began her forty-year career as a journalist, when, as a mother, she exposed the dangers of chemicals in children's sleepwear. That led to a position as a medical/consumer reporter with KERA, the PBS affiliate in Dallas, Texas, and the eventual banning of the chemicals.

Her award-winning article, "Deep Sleep," published in *D (Dallas) Magazine*, revealed the cause of an unprecedented cluster of anesthesia deaths and was the impetus for a segment on the ABC show *20/20* for which she served as a consultant.

Also, in *D Magazine*, her in-depth report "The Baby Factory" chronicled the dangerous procedures used during the birth of her second child and helped usher in a more natural approach to hospital deliveries in her home city of Fort Worth.

She won The American Cancer Society of Texas Journalist Award for her article "A Time to Die," which explained a more sensitive and honest approach to dying offered by a new and controversial program at the time—hospice.

Her video, *Shelter From the Storm of Family Violence*, which she produced in the late 1980s, helped educate the public on that hidden problem. It received an award from the Dallas Chapter of Women in Communication.

She has also served as a healthcare administrator with a major Texas healthcare system where one of her responsibilities was to implement a public education program with an emphasis on prevention. She coauthored two books with a nationally recognized physician.

Joan currently has a company that distributes the Clarity Chair, a revolutionary medical device she helped develop to improve brain function and help overcome challenges caused by injury and dysfunction.

She now adds this book on MVPS to her list of investigative reports. The text chronicles what she's learned in the effort to take back her life from the grips of MVPS. Joan knew she had to have an action plan to do that. This is hers.

Printed in Great Britain
by Amazon